MY 100 DAY DIET

MY 100 DAY DIET

A Continuous Chronological Record Depicting an Account of What I Ate

(Described in Layman's Terms)

SHIRLEY E. MALTZMAN

Writers Club Press

San Jose New York Lincoln Shanghai

MY 100 DAY DIET
A Continuous Chronological Record
Depicting an Account of What I Ate

Writers Club Press
an imprint of iUniverse.com, Inc.

For information address:
iUniverse.com, Inc.
5220 S 16th, Ste. 200
Lincoln, NE 68512
www.iuniverse.com

ISBN: 0-595-13168-9

Printed in the United States of America

To my sweet, wonderful husband, Paul, who perservered and encouraged me through this diet and still does and to Lin Sherman for her patient assistance and without whom publication of this book would not have been possible.

CONTENTS

Foreword

Nutrition is an important tool for the prevention and treatment of disease. Many attempts have been made to identify more efficient and effective means to share information and experiences that may increase awareness and promote strategies to achieve success in one of America's difficult problem over nutrition.

The author of this book shares a unique method that she designed to help permanently control overeating.

Dr. Weldon S. Lloyd, Nutritionist

My 100 Day Diet
(A layman's view of what you eat in 100 days—everything!!)

After consultation and advise from my nutritionist, I embarked on a program to lower my very high cholesterol and lose some excess pounds.

I kept a very careful and meticulous record of everything I ate and drank for more than three months and the result is this complete record (sometimes up until 2 a.m. depending on the intake). The preparation of this information took approximately two years but I feel that it was well worth the effort because it has helped me immensely. I hope it will do the same for those who read and follow this same regimen.

The method really works! Now whenever I'm eating *out* or *in* I know exactly what I am consuming; it is in my head! My cholesterol is now under control and I feel much better for it. I am not recording my food intake any more, but now I know what is best for me.

I wish to thank Dr. Weldon Lloyd, my nutritionist, who helped me greatly throughout this endeavor and who is still advising me.

The resources I utilized are as follows:
1. *Eat Smart —Guide to Diet and Nutrition* published by Random House
2. *The T-factor—Fat Gram Counter* by Jamie Pope-Cordle, M.S., R.D. and Martin Katahn, Ph.D. (one meal at a time)
3. *Guide to Cholesterol, Carbohydrate, Protein, Fat & Salt* by Merit Publications, Inc.
4. *Food Values of Portions Commonly Used* by Jean A. T. Pennington, Ph.D., R.D. (this was my bible)

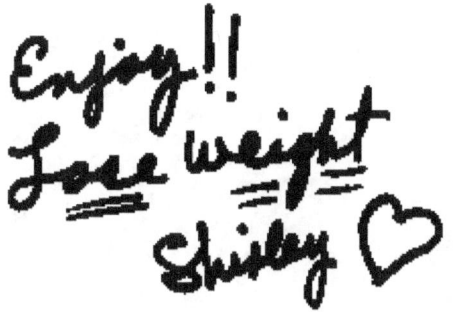

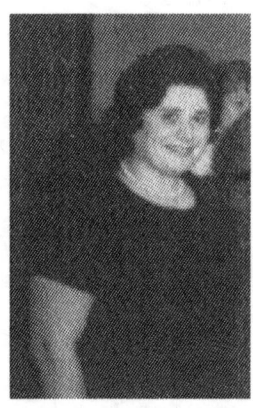
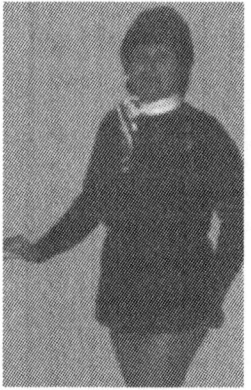

The proof—before and after!

ABBREVIATIONS

c	cup
CF	caffeine free
FF	fat free
lb	pound
LC	low calorie
LF	low fat
lrg	large
med	medium
oz	ounce
pc	piece
pkt	pocket
SF	sugar free
sl	slice
sm	small
tbsp	tablespoon
w/	with

FOODS EATEN
(by category)

BEVERAGES

apple cider
apple juice
coffee, decaffeinated
Crystal Light
daiquiri, strawberry

milk, 1%
milk, regular
milk, skim plus
orange juice
soda, apple cranberry

tea, ginseng energy
tea, herbal
yogurt flavored peach

BREADS & CEREALS

bagel, regular and mini
bread, bread
bread, black forest
bread, pita
bread, white Pepperidge
bread, potato
bread, pumpernickel (Jewish
  style)
bread, rye
cereal
Challah
cookie, sugar
cookie, fig
cookie, gingersnap
cookie, vanilla sandwich
cookie, vanilla wafer
cookie, vienna finger
crackers, fat free garlic

dinner rolls
egg noodles
English muffin
French toast (w/strawberry
  sauce)
fried dough
Graham crackers
Grainfield cereal
Knishe, Jewish style
Kellogg's Special K
lavish bread, tomato basil pita
mini bites
muffin, blueberry
noodle pudding
noodles, no yolk
oatmeal w/raisins and brown
  sugar
Oyster crackers

pasta and groats, Kasha &
  Varnislikas
pasta, ziti w/tomato sauce
pretzel
pretzel, no salt w/mustard
  cheese dip
rice cake, apple cinnamon
rice cake, low fat strawberry
rice, white
Ry-Krisps
scone, plain
scone, raisin
stuffing
vegetable crackers
Wasa Crisp

DAIRY & DAIRY SUBSTITUTES

cheese, Alpine Lace
cheese, American
cheese, hard
cheese sticks
Coffeemate Creamer
Cool Whip, light and regular
cottage cheese, fat free
cottage cheese, light

cottage cheese, low fat
cottage cheese, regular
cream cheese, light
cream cheese, regular
cream cheese, tofu
Egg Beaters
egg salad
egg, boiled

frozen dessert, 100% natural
  raspberry chill
Half & Half
ice cream, strawberry
  w/strawberry sauce
ice cream, yogurt fat free
margarine
yogurt, fat free

DESSERTS

apple pie	carrot cake	pecan pie
blueberry pie	fudge	gelatin, regular and sugar free

EATING OUT

D'Angelo's veggie delight pita	fish, fried beer battered	tortilla, spinach wrap
donut holes	McDonald's Big Mac	w/chicken cubes, vegetables,
donut, honey dipped	pizza w/green peppers	teriyaki
Dunkin Donut donut, jelly		

FRUITS

apple	dates, dried	pear
applesauce, watermelon	figs	pineapple
flavored	grapes	strawberries
banana	honey dew melon	tangerine
cantaloupe	orange, Mandarin	

MEAT, FISH, FOWL & SUBSTITUTES

bacon	hot dog, kosher	sole, fried and lightly coated
bologna, Oscar Mayer	London broil	teriyaki meat stick
lunchable	lox	tongue, deli style
chicken salad	meatballs, Italian	tunafish w/light mayonnaise
chicken, Chinese lo mein	pork, Chinese spare ribs	turkey
chicken, grilled	portabella mushroom	turkey/hamburg hamburgers
chicken breast, grilled	roast beef	veal cutlet, breaded
chicken, roasted	salmon, grilled	veggie burger
Chinese Mooshi	scrod, w/light bread crumbs	
corned beef hash	sirloin tips	

MISCELLANEOUS

candy, hard	hors d'orvres, hot dog	popcorn
candy, Juicy Twists	hors d'orvres, wrapped	potato chips
candy, red licorice	spinach	potato salad
candy, Richardson's jelly	hummus	Reuben on rye
cashews	mayonnaise	salad dressing, blue cheese
Coke, diet	manicotti, Florentine	salad dressing, ranch fat free
dressing, fat free/low sodium	onion dip (made w/sour	scallion, Chinese pancake
Fatayer, Middle Eastern dish	cream)	Sweet & Low
gelatin, mandarin orange	peanut butter	vegetable lasagne

VEGETABLES & VEGETABLE BLENDS

apple, carrot, beet, parsley mix

bean soup w/franks

beans, baked vegetarian

beans, string

cabbage

carrots

cauliflower

caesar salad

celery

coleslaw

cucumbers

green pea soup

lettuce, romaine

peas

peas, fried green

peas, sweet canned

peppers, red, yellow, green mix

pickle

potatoes, French fried w/little oil

potatoes, home fries

potatoes, roasted w/onions

potatoes, sweet

potatoes, white mashed

potatoes, mashed w/bread crumbs

salad fixings

spinach

squash

tomato sauce

tomato soup

turnip

zucchini

DAY 1

	Calories 1826 Daily	Fluids	Total Fat 60.90 Daily	Polyunsaturated Fats 20.30 Daily	Cholesterol 300 Daily	Weight Grams	Protein 47.90 Daily	Carbohydrates 264.90 Daily	Saturated Fats 18.27 Daily	Fiber 18.27 Daily	Sodium 1200 Daily	Calcium 1200 Daily	Zinc 13.0 Daily	Iron 10.0 Daily
1 tbsp Intl creamer	35	-	1.5	-	0	-	.0	6.0	.0	0.0	5.0	.0	-	.00
1 Wasa crisp bread	35	-	.0	.0	0	-	1.0	7.0	.0	1.0	55.0	.0	-	-
1 oz organic tofu cream cheese	50	-	3.0	1.0	0	-	2.0	2.0	.0	.0	-	10.0	-	.00
1 sweet potato, baked	118	-	.1	-	0	-	3.0	45.0	.0	7.0	12.0	20.0	.45	.20
½ c popcorn	55	-	1.0	-	0	-	2.0	11.0	.0	-	42.0	-	-	-
4 oz Crystal Light	3	-	.0	.0	0	-	.0	.1	-	.0	.0	.0	.00	.00
1 potato, baked	175	-	15.0	-	0	-	2.0	10.0	-	-	2.0	-	-	-
1 baked onion and spices	285	-	16.0	T	0	-	4.0	12.0	-	-	190.0	-	-	-
1 c carrots, cooked	45	-	T	.0	0	-	T	25.0	.0	-	42.0	-	-	-
1 vegetarian Portabella burger	100	-	1.5	.0	0	-	14.0	10.0	.0	3.0	390.0	4%	-	10%
¾ c beets, apples, parsley, carrots puree	36	-	20.0	-	-	-	20.0	35.0	.0	25.0	40.0	20%	0.00	10%
1 sm slice banana bread	120	-	2.0	.0	T	-	4.0	22.0	.0	-	212.0	-	-	-
DAILY TOTALS	1057	-	60.1	1.0	OK	-	52.0	185.1	OK	36.0	1202.0	OK	OK	OK

T = trace   H = high   L = low   0 = none   - none   % percent

My first day – not a good sample!

DAY 2

	Calories 1826 Daily	Fluids	Total Fat 60.90 Daily	Polyunsaturated Fats 20.30 Daily	Cholesterol 300 Daily	Weight Grams	Protein 47.90 Daily	Carbohydrates 264.90 Daily	Saturated Fats 18.27 Daily	Fiber 18.27 Daily	Sodium 1200 Daily	Calcium 1200 Daily	Zinc 13.0 Daily	Iron 10.0 Daily
8 oz decaf coffee	2	8.0	T	.0	0	-	T	T	.0	-	1.0	-	-	-
2 pkts Sweet & Low	4	-	-	-	-	1	-	-	-	-	4.0	-	-	-
1 tbsp Intl creamer	35	-	1.5	-	0	-	.0	6.0	-	.0	5.0	.0	-	0.00
18 oz water (bottle)	-	18.0	-	-	-	-	-	-	-	-	-	-	-	-
3 oz water (bottle)	-	3.0	-	-	-	-	-	-	-	-	-	-	-	-
1 oz "veggie" organic tofu cream cheese	50	-	3.0	1.0	0	-	2.0	2.0	.0	.0	220.0	10%	-	.00
1 Wasa crisp bread	35	-	.0	.0	0	-	1.0	7.0	.0	1.0	55.0	.0	-	2.00
3 slices Alpine Lace cheese	216	-	39.0	6.0	36	84	.9	20.0	10.0	.0	69.0	214.0	.93	.24
2 stalks celery	12	-	.1	.0	0	80	.3	1.5	.0	.4	35.0	14.0	5.00	.19
4 oz water	-	4.0	-	-	-	-	-	-	-	-	-	-	-	-
3 oz roast chicken	142	-	6.0	H	80	-	35.0	.0	L	.0	87.0	12.0	.00	1.70
3/4 string beans	30	-	.2	.1	0	-	1.2	4.9	.0	1.1	2.0	29.0	.23	16.00
3/4 squash cooked w/fat free margarine	23	-	.1	.1	0	-	.8	2.8	.0	.9	3.0	23.0	17.00	.30
8 oz Crystal Light	6	8.0	.0	.0	0	0	.0	.1	-	.0	0.0	.0	0.00	.00
2 tbsp ketchup	32	-	.1	.0	0	0	.3	3.8	.0	.0	300.0	3.0	0.00	.00
8 oz herbal tea	-	8.0	-	-	-	-	-	1.0	-	-	-	-	-	-
DAILY TOTALS	587	49.0	50.0	OK	116	165	41.5	49.1	10.0	3.4	781.0	295.0	23.16	20.43

T = trace   H = high   L = low   0 = none   - none   % percent

	Calories 1826 Daily	Fluids	Total Fat 60.90 Daily	Polyunsaturated Fats 20.30 Daily	Cholesterol 300 Daily	Weight Grams	Protein 47.90 Daily	Carbohydrates 264.90 Daily	Saturated Fats 18.27 Daily	Fiber 18.27 Daily	Sodium 1200 Daily	Calcium 1200 Daily	Zinc 13.0 Daily	Iron 10.0 Daily
1/2 tomato basil bagel	83	-	1.4	-	-	-	6.0	30.9	-	.6	198.0	23.0	.29	1.46
8 oz decaf coffee	2	8.0	T	0.0	0	-	T	T	.0	-	1.0	-	-	-
1 tbsp Intl creamer	35	-	1.5	-	0	-	.0	6.0	-	.0	5.0	.0	-	.00
14 oz water	-	14.0	-	-	-	-	-	-	-	-	-	-	-	-
18 oz water	-	18.0	-	-	-	-	-	-	-	-	-	-	-	-
1/2 tomato basil bagel	83	-	1.4	-	-	-	6.0	30.9	-	.6	198.0	23.0	.29	1.46
1 oz garlic & herb tofu cream cheese	80	-	.8	6.0	0	-	1.0	1.0	2.0	-	135.0	-	-	-
1 stalk celery	12	-	.1	.0	0	80	.3	1.5	.0	.4	35.0	14.0	5.00	.19
1 large carrot	45	-	T	.0	0	-	T	25.0	.0	-	42.0	-	-	-
2 pkts Sweet & Low	4	-	-	-	-	1	-	-	-	-	4.0	-	-	-
3/4 apple w/o skin	72	108.1	.4	.1	0	128	.2	.4	.1	2.9	.0	5.0	.50	.90
Break time – out for a mystery ride 1 green salad	90	-	25.0	-	-	-	.0	25.0	-	3.0	1.5	-	-	.10
4 sl mandarin orange	111	-	.1	.0	0	140	1.4	16.3	.0	.0	1.0	56.0	.08	.17
1 c ziti pasta w/ tomato sauce	238	9.3	32.9	.0	0	208	9.6	9.1	.0	.0	289.0	.0	.00	.00
8 oz decaf coffee	2	8.0	T	.0	0	0	T	T	.0	-	1.0	-	-	-
1 tbsp half/half	40	0.0	1.7	2.2	6	30	24.1	.6	1.1	.0	6.0	16.0	.08	.01
8 oz decaf coffee	2	8.0	T	.0	0	0	T	T	0.0	-	1.0	-	-	-
1 tbsp half/half	40	0.0	1.7	2.2	6	30	24.1	.6	1.1	.0	6.0	16.0	.08	.01
2 pkts Sweet & Low	4	-	-	-	-	-	T	-	-	-	4.0	-	-	-
2 pkts Sweet & Low	4	-	-	-	-	1	T	-	-	-	4.0	-	-	-
1/2 bagel	83	-	1.4	-	-	-	6.0	30.9	-	.6	198.0	23.0	.29	1.46
DAILY TOTALS	1030	173.4	68.4	OK	12	618	78.7	178.2	OK	OK	1129.5	176.0	6.61	5.76

T = trace   H = high   L = low   0 = none   - none   % percent

Day 3 – I'm getting better at this!

DAY 4

	Calories 1826 Daily	Fluids	Total Fat 60.90 Daily	Polyunsaturated Fats 20.30 Daily	Cholesterol 300 Daily	Weight Grams	Protein 47.90 Daily	Carbohydrates 264.90 Daily	Saturated Fats 18.27 Daily	Fiber 18.27 Daily	Sodium 1200 Daily	Calcium 1200 Daily	Zinc 13.0 Daily	Iron 10.0 Daily
8 oz orange juice	104	8.0	.4	.1	0	-	221.6	24.5	.1	.0	6.0	21.0	.17	1.10
Out for lunch!														
5 pork spare ribs	300	-	20.0	.6	30	-	.4	20.0	6.6	.1	100.0	.1	-	1.70
1 sm scallion pancake	60	-	20.0	.8	20	-	.1	25.0	2.2	.4	100.0	.1	-	.00
1 teriyaki stick	70	-	10.0	10.0	30	-	3.0	15.0	2.4	.6	150.0	.4	-	1.90
1 c lo mein noodles w/chicken	200	-	5.0	4.0	25	-	25.0	30.0	4.0	.8	100.0	.8	-	1.20
1/2 c mooshi Chinese	250	-	7.0	3.0	30	-	10.0	30.0	5.0	3.0	100.0	.9	-	1.10
8 oz water	-	8.0	-	-	-	-	-	-	-	-	-	-	-	-
8 oz water	-	8.0	-	-	-	-	-	-	-	-	-	-	-	-
8 oz licorice herbal tea	0	8.0	.0	.0	0	0	.0	1.0	.0	.0	.0	.0	.00	.00
3 sl Alpine Lace cheese	216	-	39.0	6.0	36	84	.9	80.0	10.0	.0	69.0	214.0	.93	.24
1 celery stalk	12	-	1.0	.0	0	80	.3	1.5	.0	.4	35.0	14.0	5.00	.19
8 oz licorice herbal tea	0	8.0	.0	.0	0	0	.0	1.0	.0	.0	.0	.0	.00	.00
8 oz water	-	8.0	-	-	-	-	-	-	-	-	-	-	-	-
DAILY TOTALS	1212	48.0	102.4	24.5	171	164	261.3	278.0	30.3	5.3	660.0	251.3	6.1	7.43

T = trace   H = high   L = low   0 = none   - none   % percent

DAY 5

	Calories 1826 Daily	Fluids	Total Fat 60.90 Daily	Polyunsaturated Fats 20.30 Daily	Cholesterol 300 Daily	Weight Grams	Protein 47.90 Daily	Carbohydrates 264.90 Daily	Saturated Fats 18.27 Daily	Fiber 18.27 Daily	Sodium 1200 Daily	Calcium 1200 Daily	Zinc 13.0 Daily	Iron 10.0 Daily
8 oz water	-	8.0	-	-	-	-	-	-	-	-	-	-	-	-
8 oz herbal tea	-	8.0	-	-	-	-	-	-	-	-	-	-	-	-
1/2 c plain cereal	110	-	.5	-	0	-	2.0	24.0	-	2.0	20.0	.0	-	5.00
1 sl Alpine Lace cheese	150	-	25.0	3.0	25	42	.6	48.0	5.0	.0	38.0	125.0	.62	.22
2 raw carrots	80	-	T	.0	0	-	T	50.0	.0	-	84.0	-	-	-
1 celery stalk	12	-	.1	.0	0	80	.3	1.5	.0	.4	3.5	14.0	5.00	.19
1 raspberry chill frozen 100% natural desert	110	8.0	.0	.0	0	-	.0	46.0	.0	.0	15.0	.0	-	.00
8 oz water	-	8.0	-	-	-	-	-	-	-	-	-	-	-	-
8 oz Crystal Light	6	8.0	-	-	-	-	-	0.1	-	-	-	-	-	-
4 oz Crystal Light	3	4.0	-	-	-	-	-	0.1	-	-	-	-	-	-
3/4 c puree blend of beets, apples, parsley, carrots	36	-	20.0	-	T	-	20.0	35.0	.0	25.0	40.0	3.0	.00	.09
1 celery stalk	12	-	.1	.0	0	80	.3	1.5	.0	.4	3.5	14.0	5.00	.19
1/2 c green, red, and yellow pepper blend	12	-	.2	.1	0	50	.4	2.7	.0	.6	2.0	3.0	.09	.63
3/4 c cooked squash	20	-	.2	.2	0	75	.9	2.9	.0	.9	4.0	18.0	20.00	.60
3/4 c FF cottage cheese	164	-	2.3	.0	0	226	28.0	6.2	1.5	19.0	918.0	138.0	.80	.32
1 "bite" roast chicken	20	-	2.0	H	10	-	10.0	.0	L	20.0	0.6	10.0	.00	1.00
2 Ry Krisps	70	-	.0	.0	0	0	2.0	14.0	.0	2.0	110.0	0.0	-	-
8 oz water	-	8.0	-	-	-	-	-	-	-	-	-	-	-	-
DAILY TOTALS	805	52.0	50.4	3.3	35	553	64.5	232.0	6.5	70.3	1238.6	325.0	31.51	8.24

T = trace   H = high   L = low   0 = none   - none   % percent

DAY 6

	Calories 1826 Daily	Fluids	Total Fat 60.90 Daily	Polyunsaturated Fats 20.30 Daily	Cholesterol 300 Daily	Weight Grams	Protein 47.90 Daily	Carbohydrates 264.90 Daily	Saturated Fats 18.27 Daily	Fiber 18.27 Daily	Sodium 1200 Daily	Calcium 1200 Daily	Zinc 13.0 Daily	Iron 10.0 Daily
1 Ry Krisp	70	-	.0	.0	0	0	2.0	14.0	.0	2.0	110.0	.0	-	-
2 tbsp tofu cream cheese	160	-	8.0	6.0	0	-	1.0	1.0	2.0	-	135.0	-	-	-
8 oz decaf coffee	2	8.0	T	.0	0	-	T	T	.0	-	1.0	-	-	-
2 pkts Sweet & Low	4	-	-	-	-	1	-	-	-	-	4.0	-	-	-
1 tbsp Intl creamer	35	-	1.5	-	0	-	.0	6.0	-	0	5.0	.0	-	.00
8 oz water	-	8.0	-	-	-	-	-	-	-	-	-	-	-	-
1/2 pickle	7	-	14.0	.0	60	-	6.0	25.0	2.0	-	728.0	.7	.00	.00
8 oz water	-	8.0	-	-	-	-	-	-	-	-	-	-	-	-
2 stalks celery	24	-	0.2	.0	0	190	6.0	1.9	.0	.8	6.9	28.0	10.00	.36
1 D'Angelo's Classic Veggie Delite on pita bread	240	-	7.0	.0	21	-	.2	.0	3.0	2.0	800.0	.0	1.00	.00
1 sl fresh pineapple (core and all!)	0	-	.0	.0	0	0	.0	65.0	.0	6.0	.0	.0	.00	3.00
1 celery stalk	12	-	.1	.0	0	80	.3	1.5	.0	.4	3.5	14.0	5.00	.19
1 oz garlic & herb tofu cream cheese	80	-	8.0	6.0	0	-	1.0	1.0	2.0	-	135.0	-	-	-
8 oz water	-	8.0	-	-	-	-	-	-	-	-	-	-	-	-
16 oz Crystal Light	12	16.0	-	-	-	-	-	.2	-	-	-	-	-	-
1-1/2 c salad greens	90	-	25.0	-	-	-	.0	25.0	-	3.0	1.5	-	-	-
2 tbsp FF ranch dressing	45	-	.0	.0	0	0	.0	11.0	.0	1.0	330.0	-	-	.10
2 c lo mein noodles w/chicken	200	-	5.0	4.0	25	-	25.0	30.0	4.0	.8	100.0	.0	.00	.00
1/2 c mooshi	250	-	7.0	3.0	30	-	10.0	30.0	5.0	3.0	100.0	.8	-	1.20
8 oz water	-	8.0	-	-	-	-	-	-	-	-	-	-	-	-
DAILY TOTALS	1231	56.0	75.8	19.0	136	271	46.1	211.6	18.0	19.0	2459.9	43.5	16.00	4.85

T = trace   H = high   L = low   0 = none   - none   % percent

3. You can contrast the gross profit margin and net profit margin of your customer with those of other companies in their industry over the previous 12 months in the Trends section.

4. The Trends section's top-right button, labeled *Industries Comparisons*, should be turned on.

5. If you haven't already, QuickBooks will ask you to choose an industry for your client. Anytime you want to update it, click the Edit icon next to Industry. Visit the North American Industry Classification System (NAICS) website for suggestions if you're unsure of which industry to choose.

6. Edit the company settings in your client's QuickBooks to alter the business location.

7. Based on companies in your client's region that have similar revenue, QuickBooks determines the industry data.

8. If QuickBooks doesn't yet have enough information for your client's industry and region, industry comparisons won't show up. As we continue to collect data, check back occasionally. TIP: To add or remove a dot from view, click on the legend of a chart. To see a data point's precise number or percentage, hover your mouse over it.

Step 4: Share a performance report.

Want to show your client what you see on the dashboard? A performance report is simple to export:

1. Create the dashboard according to your preferences. Your most recent choices will be reflected in the report. Choose the time periods you want to compare, for instance, under the Key Metrics section. At the upper right of the screen, click the Export button. The report downloads to your PC as a PDF.

Budgeting and Forecasting

What Needs to Be Done Before Using QuickBooks' Forecasting and Budgeting Features?

You must analyze your previous year's financial and fiscal statement data before preparing your QuickBooks budget and Forecast reports. To reach them, take these actions:

1. Go to the *Company* menu in QuickBooks after it is open.

2. Select the pencil-shaped icon after clicking on *My Company*.

3. Make sure the beginning month of your fiscal year is accurate before selecting the *Report Information* option.

4. Now select *Company and Financial* from the Reports menu.

5. Depending on your forecasting or budgeting requirements, choose between *Profit and Loss Detail* and *Balance Sheet Detail*.

6. Pick the most recent fiscal year from the *Dates* drop-down menu.

7. Finally, select *Refresh*. You might alternatively commit the report to memory for later use.

	Calories 1826 Daily	Fluids	Total Fat 60.90 Daily	Polyunsaturated Fats 20.30 Daily	Cholesterol 300 Daily	Weight Grams	Protein 47.90 Daily	Carbohydrates 264.90 Daily	Saturated Fats 18.27 Daily	Fiber 18.27 Daily	Sodium 1200 Daily	Calcium 1200 Daily	Zinc 13.0 Daily	Iron 10.0 Daily
16 oz water	-	16.0	-	-	-	-	-	-	-	-	-	-	-	-
8 oz decaf coffee	2	8.0	T	.0	0	-	T	T	.0	-	1.0	-	-	-
2 pkts Sweet & Low	4	-	-	-	-	1.0	-	-	-	-	4.0	-	-	-
1 tbsp Intl creamer	35	-	1.5	-	0	-	.0	6.0	-	.0	5.0	.0	-	.00
3 pieces cantaloupe	10	.2	.0	.0	0	10	30.0	10.0	-	.2	3.0	2.0	.02	.50
1 Ry Krisp	35	-	.0	.0	0	-	1.0	7.0	.0	1.0	55.0	.0	-	2.00
1 tbsp tofu cream cheese	80	-	8.0	6.0	0	-	1.0	1.0	2.0	-	135.0	-	-	-
1/2 c apple juice	97	-	.0	.1	0	82	.0	.0	.0	.0	30.0	.0	.00	.00
2 tbsp tofu cream cheese	80	-	8.0	6.0	0	-	1.0	1.0	2.0	-	135.0	-	-	-
10 vegetable crackers	150	-	-	-	0	-	2.0	19.0	1.0	1.0	290.0	2.0	-	1.00
8 oz water	-	8.0	-	-	-	-	-	-	-	-	-	-	-	-
1 carrot	40	-	T	.0	0	-	T	25.0	.0	-	42.0	-	-	-
Out for dinner 1 serving fish (sole) & chips (thin coated)	440	-	25.0	.0	0	198	20.0	35.0	.0	.0	640.0		-	-
2 c French Fries (little oil)	300	19.0	18.3	8.8	0	100	4.0	40.0	4.5	.0	216.0	20.0	38.00	7.60
1/4 c coleslaw	61	36.4	6.0	.0	18	50	1.4	6.0	.0	.0	120.0	22.0	10.00	-
3 c decaf coffee	6	24.0	T	.0	0	-	T	T	T	.0	3.0	-	-	-
1 tbsp Intl creamer	35	25.0	2.9	.1	9	100	5.5	7.0	.1	9.0	95.0	100.0	1.00	7.50
1 green salad	90	25.0	-	-	-	-	-	25.0	-	3.0	1.5	-	-	0.10
6 pkts Sweet & Low	6	-	-	-	-	3	-	-	12.0	-	-	-	-	-
1 tbsp Key Lime pie	80	20.1	5.4	.0	0	90	2.3	30.2	.0	.0	100.0	9.0	16.00	1.00
1 tbsp honey dijon dressing	25	1.1	4.4	2.2	0	7	.0	0.2	1.0	-	40.0	.0	.00	.00
DAILY TOTALS	1576	182.8	79.5	23.2	27	641	68.2	212.4	26.6	14.2	1915.5	155.0	65.02	19.70

T = trace   H = high   L = low   0 = none   - none   % percent

DAY 8
On vacation!

	Calories 1826 Daily	Fluids	Total Fat 60.90 Daily	Polyunsaturated Fats 20.30 Daily	Cholesterol 300 Daily	Weight Grams	Protein 47.90 Daily	Carbohydrates 264.90 Daily	Saturated Fats 18.27 Daily	Fiber 18.27 Daily	Sodium 1200 Daily	Calcium 1200 Daily	Zinc 13.0 Daily	Iron 10.0 Daily
Out for Breakfast														
8 oz cranberry juice	102	160.6	.0	.0	0	187	.0	26.2	.0	.0	6.0	9.0	.70	.17
1/2 French toast w/strawberry sauce	150	46.2	3.9	-	-	85	6.4	26.8	-	-	220.0	54.0	.80	1.00
1 bagel	163	-	2.8	-	-	-	12.0	61.0	-	1.2	300.0	46.0	.50	3.00
1 tbsp cream cheese light	62	18.3	4.7	.1	16	28	2.9	1.8	2.8	.0	160.0	38.0	.21	.40
1/2 c cottage cheese	164	-	2.3	.0	0	226	28.0	6.2	1.5	19.0	918.0	138.0	.80	.32
1/2 c cantaloupe and fresh pineapple	80	.6	0.0	.0	0	30	90.0	30.0	-	.6	9.0	6.0	.08	.12
3 c decaf coffee	6	24.0	T	.0	0	-	T	T	.0	-	3.0	-	-	-
4 pkts Sweet & Low	6	-	-	-	-	-	-	6.0	-	-	-	-	-	-
3 packets Half & Half	120	.0	2.1	6.8	18	90	88.3	1.8	2.2	.0	-	-	-	-
Thanksgiving Dinner														
3 c water	-	24.0	-	-	-	-	-	-	-	-	-	-	-	
2 sm sweet potatoes	183	152.1	.4	.2	0	200	3.3	42.3	.1	-	107.0	44.0	.36	1.77
1 green salad	90	25.0	-	-	-	-	-	25.0	-	3.0	1.5	-	-	.10
1/4 c mashed potatoes w/margarine	111	80.1	4.4	1.3	2	105	2.0	17.5	1.1	.0	309.0	27.0	0.29	.28
3/4 c stuffing	416	122.8	25.6	.0	0	200	8.8	39.4	13.1	-	1008.0	80.0	-	2.00
3 slices turkey breast	157	66.3	3.2	.9	69	100	29.9	.0	1.0	.0	64.0	19.0	2.04	.02
1 sm slice roast beef	200	25.0	20.2	.1	58	50	18.0	.0	6.3	.0	35.0	7.0	6.00	1.42
1/2 c squash	23	-	.1	.1	0	-	.8	2.8	0.0	.9	3.0	23.0	17.00	.30
3 c decaf herbal tea	-	24.0	-	-	-	-	-	3.0	-	-	-	-	-	-
2 pkts Sweet & Low	4	-	-	-	-	1	-	-	-	-	4.0	-	-	-
1 slice pecan pie	431	20.1	23.6	-	-	103	5.3	52.8	3.3	-	228.0	48.0	-	2.90
1 slice carrot cake	187	1.0	4.0	-	0	44	1.6	36.1	-	-	253.0	62.0	.09	.62
DAILY TOTALS	2655	790.1	97.3	9.5	163	1449	297.3	372.7	37.4	24.7	3628.5	601.0	28.87	14.42

T = trace   H = high   L = low   0 = none   - none   % percent

DAY 9
Vacation Day 2

	Calories 1826 Daily	Fluids	Total Fat 60.90 Daily	Polyunsaturated Fats 20.30 Daily	Cholesterol 300 Daily	Weight Grams	Protein 47.90 Daily	Carbohydrates 264.90 Daily	Saturated Fats 18.27 Daily	Fiber 18.27 Daily	Sodium 1200 Daily	Calcium 1200 Daily	Zinc 13.0 Daily	Iron 10.0 Daily
Out for breakfast														
10 crackers	150	-	-	-	0	-	2.0	19.00	1.0	1.0	290.0	2.0	-	6.00
1 c cantaloupe	57	143.6	.4	-	-	160.00	1.4	13.40	-	.5	14.0	17.0	.250	.34
1 c cantaloupe (again!)	57	143.6	.4	-	-	160.00	1.4	13.40	-	.5	14.0	17.0	.250	.34
1/2 c cottage cheese	164	-	2.3	.0	0	226.00	28.0	6.20	1.5	19.0	918.0	138.0	.800	.32
1 bagel	163	-	2.8	-	-	-	12.0	61.00	-	.12	300.0	46.0	.500	3.00
3/4 c oatmeal w/raisins & brown sugar	134	25.0	1.6	-	-	35.00	3.9	26.00	-	-	181.0	100.0	1.000	4.50
16 oz decaf coffee	4	16.0	T	.0	0	-	T	T	.0	1.0	2.0	-	-	-
2 pkts Sweet & Low	4	-	-	-	-	1.00	.0	-	-	-	4.0	-	-	-
1 tbsp Intl creamer	35	-	1.5	-	0	-	.0	6.00	-	.0	5.0	.0	-	.00
And for dinner too!														
16 oz decaf coffee	4	16.0	T	0.0	0	-	T	T	.0	-	2.0	-	-	-
2 pkts Sweet & Low	4	-	-	-	-	1.00	0	-	-	-	4.0	-	-	-
1 tbsp Intl creamer	35	-	1.5	-	0	-	.0	6.00	-	.0	5.0	.0	-	.00
1 strawberry non-alcoholic daiquiri	262	91.7	2.6	.5	0	141.00	.6	39.90	1.2	-	100.0	10.0	.116	.31
1 c cooked vegetable blend - zucchini, squash, carrots	70	100.1	.4	.2	0	1.62	4.2	14.12	.0	4.0	122.0	22.0	.340	.86
2 dinner rolls	116	-	2.0	-	15	56.00	4.0	28.00	-	-	170.0	-	-	-
2 pats margarine	150	-	22.0	16.0	0	-	-	-	4.0	-	5.0	-	-	-
1 serving scrod w/bread crumbs	347	-	21.7	-	49	156.00	26.4	11.40	-	-	312.0	91.0	-	1.70
8 oz water	-	8.0	-	-	-	-	-	-	-	-	-	-	-	-
DAILY TOTALS	1756	544.0	59.2	16.7	64	937.62	83.9	244.42	7.7	26.12	2448.0	443.0	3.256	17.37

T = trace   H = high   L = low   0 = none   - none   % percent

	Calories 1826 Daily	Fluids	Total Fat 60.90 Daily	Polyunsaturated Fats 20.30 Daily	Cholesterol 300 Daily	Weight Grams	Protein 47.90 Daily	Carbohydrates 264.90 Daily	Saturated Fats 18.27 Daily	Fiber 18.27 Daily	Sodium 1200 Daily	Calcium 1200 Daily	Zinc 13.0 Daily	Iron 10.0 Daily
1 bagel	163	-	2.8	-	-	-	12.0	61.0	-	.12	300.0	46.0	.50	3.00
1 tbsp light cream cheese	62	18.3	4.7	.1	16	28	29.0	1.8	2.8	.00	160.0	38.0	.21	.40
1/2 c cottage cheese	164	-	2.3	.0	0	226	28.0	6.2	1.5	19.00	918.0	138.0	.80	.32
8 oz orange juice	111	219.0	.5	.1	0	248	1.7	25.8	.1	-	2.0	28.0	.13	.50
1/2 c home fries	158	19.0	8.3	3.8	0	50	2.0	20.0	2.5	-	108.0	10.0	.19	.38
24 oz decaf coffee	6	24.0	T	.0	0	-	T	T	.0	-	3.0	-	-	-
2 pkts Sweet & Low	4	-	-	-	-	1	-	-	4.0	-	-	-	-	-
1 tbsp Intl creamer	35	-	1.5	-	0	-	.0	6.0	-	.00	5.0	.0	-	.00
3/4 c oatmeal w/raisins & brown sugar	134	2.5	1.6	-	-	35	3.9	26.0	-	-	181.0	100.0	1.00	4.50
2 French toast sticks w/1 tbsp strawberry sauce	150	46.2	3.9	-	-	85	6.4	26.8	-	-	220.0	54.0	.08	1.00
1 very lean Reuben on rye sandwich	512	-	31.4	-	105	194	30.1	39.4	-	-	1224.0	237.0	5.23	.43
8 oz water	-	8.0	-	-	-	-	-	-	-	-	-	-	-	-
1 c french fries	300	19.0	18.3	8.8	0	100	4.0	40.0	4.5	.00	216.0	20.0	.38	.76
1 caesar green salad	160	-	.6	-	-	136	1.15	28.2	-	-	636.0	48.0		.82
1 tbsp dressing	25	1.1	4.4	2.2	0	7	.0	.2	1.0	-	40.0	.0	.00	.00
8 oz diet soda	-	8.0	-	-	-	-	-	-	-	-	4.0	-	-	-
2 dinner rolls	116	-	2.0	-	15	56	4.0	28.0	-	-	170.0	-	-	-
1 pat margarine	75	-	12.0	8.0	0	-	-	-	2.0	-	3.0	-	-	-
DAILY TOTALS	2157	365.1	94.3	23.0	136	1166	122.25	309.4	18.4	19.12	4190.0	719.0	8.52	12.11

WOW!

T = trace   H = high   L = low   0 = none   - none   % percent

DAY 11

	Calories 1826 Daily	Fluids	Total Fat 60.90 Daily	Polyunsaturated Fats 20.30 Daily	Cholesterol 300 Daily	Weight Grams	Protein 47.90 Daily	Carbohydrates 264.90 Daily	Saturated Fats 18.27 Daily	Fiber 18.27 Daily	Sodium 1200 Daily	Calcium 1200 Daily	Zinc 13.0 Daily	Iron 10.0 Daily
Out for brunch														
1 c orange juice	111	8.0	.5	.1	0	248	1.7	25.8	.1	-	2.0	28.0	.13	.50
1 bagel	163	-	2.8	-	-	-	12.0	61.0	-	.12	300.0	46.0	.50	3.00
3 c decaf coffee	6	24.0	T	.0	0	-	T	T	.0	-	3.0	-	-	-
2 pkts Sweet & Low	4	-	-	-	-	1	-	-	4.0	-	-	-	-	-
1 tbsp Intl creamer	35	-	1.5	-	0	-	.0	6.0	-	.00	5.0	.0	-	.00
1 c tuna fish w/light mayonnaise	800	129.5	29.0	18.5	37	405	65.0	38.6	6.4	-	1600.0	70.0	2.30	4.08
vegetable salad: lettuce, cukes, green and red peppers	200	-	.1	-	-	200	2.3	45.3	-	-	800.0	89.0	-	.10
1 thin sl homemade blueberry pie	175	-	5.5	-	-	50	1.0	20.1	1.0	-	100.0	3.0	-	.20
2 c fresh fruit: pineapple, cantaloupe, honeydew melon	114	4.0	.8	-	-	280	2.8	24.8	-	.10	28.0	24.0	.50	.68
1 tbsp dressing	25	1.1	4.4	2.2	0	7	.0	.2	1.0	-	40.0	.0	.00	.00
1 tbsp stuffing	20	-	10.1	.0	0	20	1.0	20.1	2.5	-	25.0	6.0	-	.10
8 oz tea	0	8.0	-	-	-	-	-	1.0	-	-	-	-	-	-
1/2 c carrots	45	-	T	.0	0	-	T	25.0	.0	-	42.0	-	-	-
1/2 c celery	12	-	1.0	.0	0	80	.3	1.1	.0	.40	35.0	14.0	5.00	.19
8 oz Crystal Light	6	8.0	.0	.0	0	0	.0	.1	-	.00	.0	.0	.00	.00
DAILY TOTALS	1716	182.6	55.7	20.8	37	1291	86.1	269.1	15.0	.62	2980.0	280.0	8.43	8.85

T = trace   H = high   L = low   0 = none   - none   % percent

DAY 12

	Calories 1826 Daily	Fluids	Total Fat 60.90 Daily	Polyunsaturated Fats 20.30 Daily	Cholesterol 300 Daily	Weight Grams	Protein 47.90 Daily	Carbohydrates 264.90 Daily	Saturated Fats 18.27 Daily	Fiber 18.27 Daily	Sodium 1200 Daily	Calcium 1200 Daily	Zinc 13.0 Daily	Iron 10.0 Daily
8 oz water	-	8.0	-	-	-	-	-	-	-	-	-	-	-	-
8 oz decaf coffee	2	8.0	T	.0	0	-	T	T	.0	-	1.0	-	-	-
2 pkts Sweet & Low	4	-	-	-	-	1	-	-	4.0	-	-	-	-	-
1 tbsp Intl creamer	35	-	1.5	-	0	-	.0	6.0	-	.0	5.0	.0	-	.00
2 Ry-Krisp crackers	70	-	.0	.0	0	-	2.0	14.0	.0	1.0	110.0	.0	-	4.00
1 FF yogurt	120	-	.0	.0	5	0	5.0	24.0	.0	.0	75.0	15.0	-	.00
1 apple, medium	85	-	T	.0	0	-	T	25.0	.0	-	42.0	-	-	-
1 carrot	40	-	T	.0	0	-	T	25.0	.0	-	42.0	-	-	-
2 celery stalks	24	-	1.1	.0	0	160	.9	2.9	.0	.8	6.9	28.0	10.00	28.00
3/4 c cottage cheese	185	-	4.9	.0	0	300	35.0	9.9	2.9	22.0	1000.0	150.0	.90	.62
1 tbsp tofu cream cheese	80	-	8.0	6.0	0	-	1.0	1.0	2.0	.0	135.0	-	-	-
8 oz water	-	8.0	-	-	-	-	-	-	-	-	-	-	-	-
green salad w/carrots and celery (no drsg)	120	30.0	-		-	-	-	35.0	-	6.0	2.1	-	-	1.00
1 c stuffing	500	-	.0	.0	0	300	9.2	50.0	22.1	-	1000.0	90.0	-	2.5
8 oz diet soda	-	8.0	-	-	-	-	-	-	-	-	4.0	-	-	-
1 sm sl turkey (dark) 2 med sl turkey (white)	180	-	6.5	1.9	100	150	32.0	.0	2.1	.0	68.0	22.0	3.01	.03
1 sm sl potato bread	80	-	1.0	-	8	35	2.0	20.0	-	-	65.0	-	-	-
2 pkts Sweet & Low	4	-	-	-	-	1	-	-	4.0	-	-	-	-	-
8 oz licorice tea	-	8.0	-	-	-	-	-	1.0	-	-	-	-	-	-
DAILY TOTALS	1529	70	23.0	7.9	113	947	87.1	213.8	37.1	29.8	2556.0	305.0	13.91	36.15

T = trace   H = high   L = low   0 = none   - none   % percent

DAY 13

	Calories 1826 Daily	Fluids	Total Fat 60.90 Daily	Polyunsaturated Fats 20.30 Daily	Cholesterol 300 Daily	Weight Grams	Protein 47.90 Daily	Carbohydrates 264.90 Daily	Saturated Fats 18.27 Daily	Fiber 18.27 Daily	Sodium 1200 Daily	Calcium 1200 Daily	Zinc 13.0 Daily	Iron 10.0 Daily
8 oz decaf coffee	2	8.0	T	.0	0	-	T	T	.0	-	1.0	-	-	-
2 pkts Sweet & Low	4	-	-	-	-	1	-	-	4.0	-	-	-	-	-
1 tbsp Intl creamer	35	-	1.5	-	0	-	.0	6.00	-	.0	5.0	.0	-	.00
1 tangerine	37	73.6	.2	.0	0	84	.5	9.40	.0	-	1.0	12.0	-	.18
2 Ry-Krisp crackers	70	-	.0	.0	0	-	2.0	14.00	.0	1.0	110.0	.0	-	4.00
2 tbsp tofu cream cheese	80	-	8.0	6.0	0	-	1.0	1.00	2.0	-	135.0	-	-	-
1 raw carrot	40	-	T	.0	0	-	T	25.00	.0	-	42.0	-	-	-
3 oz hard cheese	310	33.9	24.9	.1	71	74	18.3	.24	15.9	.0	380.0	400.0	.74	.14
18 oz water	-	8.0	-	-	-	-	-	-	-	-	-	-	-	-
1 potato, baked	145	117.7	.2	.1	0	156	3.1	33.60	.0	-	8.0	8.0	.45	.55
green salad w/carrots	120	30.0	-	-	-	-	-	35.00	-	6.0	2.1	-	-	1.00
8 oz licorice tea	-	8.0	-	-	-	-	-	-	-	-	-	-	-	-
1 c cooked vegetables cauliflower, carrots, snow peas	60	-	.0	-	0	-	2.0	6.00	.0	2.0	25.0	2.0	-	2.00
1 raw carrot	40	-	T	.0	0	-	T	25.00	.0	-	42.0	-	-	-
1/2 c bagel (reg)	83	-	1.4	-	-	-	6.0	30.90	-	.6	198.0	23.0	.29	1.46
2 tbsp tofu cream cheese	80	-	8.0	6.0	0	-	1.0	1.00	2.0	-	135.0	-	-	-
8 oz water	-	8.0	-	-	-	-	-	-	-	-	-	-	-	-
8 oz tea	-	8.0	-	-	-	-	-	-	-	-	-	-	-	-
DAILY TOTALS	1106	295.2	44.2	12.2	71	315	33.9	187.14	23.9	9.6	1084.1	445.0	1.48	9.33

T = trace   H = high   L = low   0 = none   - none   % percent

DAY 14

	Calories 1826 Daily	Fluids	Total Fat 60.90 Daily	Polyunsaturated Fats 20.30 Daily	Cholesterol 300 Daily	Weight Grams	Protein 47.90 Daily	Carbohydrates 264.90 Daily	Saturated Fats 18.27 Daily	Fiber 18.27 Daily	Sodium 1200 Daily	Calcium 1200 Daily	Zinc 13.0 Daily	Iron 10.0 Daily
8 oz decaf coffee	2	8.0	T	.0	0	-	T	T	.0	-	1.0	-	-	-
1 tbsp Intl creamer	35	-	1.5	-	0	-	.0	6.0	-	.0	5.0	.0	-	.00
2 pkts Sweet & Low	4	-	-	-	-	1	-	-	4.0	-	-	-	-	-
2 Ry Krisps	70	-	.0	.0	0	-	2.0	14.0	.0	1.0	110.0	.0	-	4.00
2 tbsp tofu cream cheese	80	-	8.0	6.0	0	-	1.0	1.0	2.0	-	135.0	-	-	-
1 banana	105	84.7	.6	.1	0	114	1.2	26.7	.2	1.6	1.0	7.0	.19	.35
1 container FF peach yogurt	110	-	.0	.0	5	0	5.0	23.0	.0	.0	75.0	15.0	.00	.00
1 glass CF diet soda	-	8.0	-	-	-	-	-	-	-	-	4.0	-	-	-
8 oz herbal tea (fruit)	-	8.0	-	-	-	-	-	-	-	-	-	-	-	-
8 oz herbal tea (fruit)	-	8.0	-	-	-	-	-	-	-	-	-	-	-	-
2 veggie burgers	200	-	4.0	-	0	-	24.0	20.0	.0	6.0	960.0	8.0	-	.20
1 c mixed vegetables onions, zucchini, cauliflower, carrots	120	-	.0	-	0	-	2.0	6.0	.0	2.0	25.0	2.0	-	2.00
1 large salad	150	-	-	-	-	-	-	50.0	-	8.0	3.3	-	-	2.00
1- 1/4 oz (bite size) Kellogg's Frosted Mini Flakes	120	-	5.0	-	0	-	3.0	28.0	.0	3.0	.0	.0	.06	.06
8 oz herbal tea	-	8.0	-	-	-	-	-	1.0	-	-	-	-	-	-
DAILY TOTALS	996	124.7	19.1	6.1	5	115	38.2	175.7	6.2	21.6	1319.3	32.0	.25	8.61

T = trace   H = high   L = low   0 = none   - none   % percent

DAY 15

	Calories 1826 Daily	Fluids	Total Fat 60.90 Daily	Polyunsaturated Fats 20.30 Daily	Cholesterol 300 Daily	Weight Grams	Protein 47.90 Daily	Carbohydrates 264.90 Daily	Saturated Fats 18.27 Daily	Fiber 18.27 Daily	Sodium 1200 Daily	Calcium 1200 Daily	Zinc 13.0 Daily	Iron 10.0 Daily
4 oz orange juice w/calcium	75	4.0	.2	.1	0	128	1.5	12.9	.1	-	1.0	1.4	.60	.25
8 oz decaf coffee	2	8.0	T	.0	0	-	T	T	.0	-	1.0	-	-	-
1 tbsp Intl creamer	35	-	1.5	-	0	-	.0	6.0	-	.00	5.0	.0	-	.00
2 pkts Sweet & Low	4	-	-	-	-	1	-	-	4.0	-	-	-	-	-
1 tbsp tofu cream cheese	40	-	8.0	6.0	0	-	1.0	1.0	2.0	-	135.0	-	-	-
1 tomato basil bagel	163	-	2.8	-	-	-	12.0	61.0	-	.12	300.0	46.0	.50	3.00
1 tbsp tofu cream cheese	80	-	8.0	6.0	0	-	1.0	1.0	2.0	-	135.0	-	-	-
1 raw carrot	40	-	T	.0	0	-	T	25.0	.0	-	42.0	-	-	-
6 tbsp humus	90	-	75.0	-	0	-	6.0	12.0	-	3.00	310.0	.0	-	.60
20 (approx) vegetable crackers	150	-	.0	-	0	-	4.0	9.0	.0	4.00	50.0	4.0	-	2.00
8 oz water	-	8.0	-	-	-	-	-	-	-	-	-	-	-	-
1-1/2 c mixed vegs zucchini, carrots, cauliflower, onions, pea pods	150	-	.0	-	0	-	4.0	9.0	.0	4.00	50.0	4.0	-	2.00
1 veggie burger	100	-	4.0	-	0	-	14.0	10.0	.0	3.00	330.0	4.0	-	.10
1/2 sl fresh pineapple	20	.0	.0	.0	0	0	25.0	25.0	.0	3.00	.0	.0	.00	2.00
8 oz Crystal Light	6	8.0	-	-	-	-	-	.2	-	-	-	-	-	-
8 oz herbal tea	-	8.0	-	-	-	-	-	1.0	-	-	4.0	-	-	-
8 oz water	-	8.0	-	-	-	-	-	-	-	-	-	-	-	-
DAILY TOTALS	955	44.0	99.5	12.1	0	129	68.5	173.1	8.1	17.12	1363.0	59.4	1.10	9.95

T = trace   H = high   L = low   0 = none   - none   % percent

DAY 16

	Calories 1826 Daily	Fluids	Total Fat 60.90 Daily	Polyunsaturated Fats 20.30 Daily	Cholesterol 300 Daily	Weight Grams	Protein 47.90 Daily	Carbohydrates 264.90 Daily	Saturated Fats 18.27 Daily	Fiber 18.27 Daily	Sodium 1200 Daily	Calcium 1200 Daily	Zinc 13.0 Daily	Iron 10.0 Daily
8 oz Skim "Plus" milk	110	8.0	.0	-	4	-	11.0	17.0	.0	.0	-	-	-	-
2 boxes Special K	140	-	.0	-	0	-	8.0	32.0	.0	2.0	-	-	-	-
8 oz water	-	8.0	-	-	-	-	-	-	-	-	-	-	-	-
4 oz orange juice w/calcium	75	4.0	.2	.1	0	128	1.5	12.9	.1	-	1.0	1.4	.60	.25
1 tbsp pumpkin, crushed pineapple, eggs, flour, sugar blend sweet potato square	150	-	20.0	2.0	120	-	2.1	32.0	3.0	1.0	300.0	-	.10	.20
3 squares veg blend: zucchini, broccoli, eggs, onions, grated pototato	200	-	30.0	2.0	200	-	2.1	25.0	.4	1.0	200	.0	1.0	1.0
8 oz water	-	8.0	-	-	-	-	-	-	-	-	-	-	-	-
8 oz herbal tea	-	8.0	-	-	-	-	-	1.0	-	-	-	-	-	-
1 sl challah	95	-	.6	-	-	45	2.5	20.5	-	-	113.0	4.1	-	.70
1/2 c LF cottage cheese	164	-	2.3	.0	0	226	28.0	6.2	1.5	.0	918.0	138.0	.80	.32
1 baked potato	145	-	.2	.1	0	156	3.1	33.6	.0	-	8.0	8.0	.45	.55
1 sl fresh pineapple	40	.0	.0	.0	0	0	50.0	50.0	.0	6.0	.0	.0	.00	4.00
8 oz herbal tea	-	8.0	-	-	-	-	1.0	-	-	-	-	-	-	-
2 pkts Sweet & Low	4	-	-	-	-	1	-	-	4.0	-	-	-	-	-
8 oz water	-	8.0	-	-	-	-	-	-	-	-	-	-	-	-
DAILY TOTALS	1123	52.0	53.3	4.2	324	556	108.3	230.2	9.0	10.0	1540.0	151.5	2.95	7.02

T = trace   H = high   L = low   0 = none   - none   % percent

	Calories 1826 Daily	Fluids	Total Fat 60.90 Daily	Polyunsaturated Fats 20.30 Daily	Cholesterol 300 Daily	Weight Grams	Protein 47.90 Daily	Carbohydrates 264.90 Daily	Saturated Fats 18.27 Daily	Fiber 18.27 Daily	Sodium 1200 Daily	Calcium 1200 Daily	Zinc 13.0 Daily	Iron 10.0 Daily
2 raw carrots	80	-	T	.0	0	-	T	50.0	.0	-	84.0	-	-	-
4 oz orange juice	75	4.0	.2	.1	0	128	1.5	12.9	.1	-	1.0	1.4	.60	.25
1 large bagel	185	-	4.8	-	-	-	24.0	122.0	-	.24	600.0	8.5	.90	7.20
2 tbsp cream cheese	99	-	9.9	-	31	-	1.1	7.0	6.2	.00	84.0	20.0	-	.10
1/2 c watermelon applesauce	80	-	.0	-	0	-	.0	20.0	-	1.00	20.0	-	-	-
Dinner out! 1 big pretzel w/mustard and no salt cheese dip	111	.7	1.0	.0	0	28	3.6	23.4	.0	.00	500.0	14.0	.30	.80
1 large green salad	150	-	-	-	-	-	-	50.0	-	8.00	3.3	-	-	2.00
3 sm rolls (used with cheese dip)	200	-	4.0	-	30	8.8	8.0	56.0	-	-	340.0	-	-	-
1 tbsp blue cheese dressing	25	1.1	4.4	2.2	0	7	.0	.2	1.0	-	40.0	.0	.00	.00
1 baked potato	145	-	.2	.1	0	156	3.1	33.6	.0	-	8.0	8.0	.45	55
6 oz grilled chicken	320	-	16.0	-	80	174	24.0	16.0	.0	10.00	300.0	18.0	1.80	-
1 c cooked carrots	80	-	T	.0	0	-	T	50.0	.0	-	84.0	-	-	-
8 oz decaf coffee	2	8.0	T	.0	0	-	T	T	.0	-	1.0	-	-	-
1 tbsp 1% milk	25	1.0	3.0	.0	8	-	2.0	4.0	.4	.10	40.0	1.5	-	.10
1 tbsp strawberry sauce	92	11.9	.8	-	0	38	.9	23.5	.4	.00	106.0	32.5	.60	15.00
1 lrg piece fried dough	56	2.0	30.0	.0	0	80	.0	5.0	.0	2.00	.0	.0	.00	.00
24 oz diet Coke	320	24.0	.0	.0	0	360	.0	8.0	.0	.00	2.0	.0	.00	.00
DAILY TOTALS	2045	52.7	74.3	2.4	149	979.8	68.2	481.6	8.1	21.34	2213.3	103.9	4.65	26.00

T = trace   H = high   L = low   0 = none   - none   % percent

DAY 18

	Calories 1826 Daily	Fluids	Total Fat 60.90 Daily	Polyunsaturated Fats 20.30 Daily	Cholesterol 300 Daily	Weight Grams	Protein 47.90 Daily	Carbohydrates 264.90 Daily	Saturated Fats 18.27 Daily	Fiber 18.27 Daily	Sodium 1200 Daily	Calcium 1200 Daily	Zinc 13.0 Daily	Iron 10.0 Daily
4 oz orange juice	75	4.0	.2	.1	0	128	1.5	12.9	.10	-	1.0	1.4	.60	.25
8 oz decaf coffee	2	8.0	T	.0	0	-	T	T	.00	-	1.0	-	-	-
1 tbsp Intl creamer	35	-	1.5	-	0	-	.0	6.0	-	.0	5.0	.0	-	.00
2 pkts Sweet & Low	4	-	-	-	-	1	-	-	4.00	-	-	-	-	-
16 oz water	-	16.0	-	-	-	-	-	-	-	-	-	-	-	-
1 sl banana bread	250	.0	11.0	.0	0	-	3.0	36.0	.00	.0	290.0	.0	.00	.93
1/4 c raw cashews	326	.1	26.4	4.4	0	56	8.8	18.6	41.20	.0	8.0	26.0	2.50	2.40
1 sl challah	95	-	.6	-	-	45	2.5	20.5	-	-	113.0	4.1	-	.70
2 tbsp tofu cream cheese	80	-	8.0	6.0	0	-	1.0	1.0	2.00	-	135.0	-	-	-
2 turkey/hamburg burgers (reg size)	1172	46.7	39.9	1.0	128	56	40.2	18.8	3.00	3.1	900.0	62.0	-	5.80
1 c green pea soup	126	68.6	.4	.2	0	160	8.2	22.8	.00	6.0	140.0	38.0	.15	-
12 oz Crystal Light	10	12.0	-	-	-	-	-	.4	-	-	-	-	-	-
8 oz herbal tea	-	8.0	-	-	-	-	-	1.0	-	-	-	-	-	-
8 oz water	-	8.0	-	-	-	-	-	-	-	-	-	-	-	-
2 pkts Sweet & Low	4	-	-	-	-	1	-	-	4.00	-	-	-	-	-
DAILY TOTALS	2179	171.4	88.0	11.7	128	447	65.2	138.0	17.22	9.1	1593.0	131.5	3.25	10.08

T = trace   H = high   L = low   0 = none   - none   % percent

DAY 19

	Calories 1826 Daily	Fluids	Total Fat 60.90 Daily	Polyunsaturated Fats 20.30 Daily	Cholesterol 300 Daily	Weight Grams	Protein 47.90 Daily	Carbohydrates 264.90 Daily	Saturated Fats 18.27 Daily	Fiber 18.27 Daily	Sodium 1200 Daily	Calcium 1200 Daily	Zinc 13.0 Daily	Iron 10.0 Daily
8 oz decaf coffee	2	8.0	T	.0	0	-	T	T	.0	-	1.0	-	-	-
2 pkts Sweet & Low	4	-	-	-	-	1	-	-	4.0	-	-	-	-	-
1 tbsp Intl creamer	35	-	1.5	-	0	-	.0	6.0	-	.0	5.0	.0	-	.00
8 oz water	-	8.0	-	-	-	-	-	-	-	-	-	-	-	-
1 sl banana bread	250	.0	11.0	.0	0	-	3.0	36.0	.0	.0	290.0	.0	.00	.93
1/2 c tuna fish salad	383	129.5	19.0	8.5	27	205	32.9	19.2	3.2	-	824.0	35.0	1.15	2.04
2 sl American cheese	420	-	40.0	8.0	90	100	12.3	95.0	10.0	.0	85.0	310.0	1.20	.75
1 sl pineapple	40	.0	.0	.0	0	0	50.0	50.0	.0	6.0	.0	.0	.00	4.00
1 carrot	40	-	T	.0	0	-	T	25.0	.0	-	42.0	-	-	-
1 c Campbell's Tomato soup	160	-	.0	-	0	-	2.0	36.0	.0	4.0	900.0	4.0	-	8.00
4 oz 1% milk	55	4.0	1.4	-	12	-	4.0	9.0	1.0	.0	-	25.0	-	.00
3 sm rolls	180	-	3.0	-	30	70	8.0	30.0	-	-	220.0	-	-	-
1/2 c tuna fish salad	383	129.5	19.0	8.5	27	205	32.9	19.2	3.2	-	824.0	35.0	1.15	2.04
1/2 c egg salad	225	-	15.0	.0	375	-	20.0	2.0	1.1	.0	29.0	1.0	.50	.36
16 oz tea	-	16.0	-	-	-	-	-	2.0	-	-	-	-	-	-
2 pkts Sweet & Low	4	-	-	-	-	1	-	-	4.0	-	-	-	-	-
8 oz water	-	8.0	-	-	-	-	-	-	-	-	-	-	-	-
DAILY TOTALS	2181	330.0	109.9	25.0	561	582	165.1	329.4	26.5	10.0	3320.0	410.0	4.00	18.12

T = trace   H = high   L = low   0 = none   - none   % percent

DAY 20

	Calories 1826 Daily	Fluids	Total Fat 60.90 Daily	Polyunsaturated Fats 20.30 Daily	Cholesterol 300 Daily	Weight Grams	Protein 47.90 Daily	Carbohydrates 264.90 Daily	Saturated Fats 18.27 Daily	Fiber 18.27 Daily	Sodium 1200 Daily	Calcium 1200 Daily	Zinc 13.0 Daily	Iron 10.0 Daily
8 oz decaf coffee	2	8.0	T	.0	0	-	T	T	.0	-	1.0	-	-	-
2 pkts Sweet & Low	4	-	-	-	-	1	-	-	4.0	-	-	-	-	-
1 tbsp Intl creamer	35	-	1.5	-	0	-	.0	6.0	-	.00	5.0	.00	-	.00
17 potato chips	150	-	10.0	-	0	-	2.0	14.0	-	.00	150.0	.00	-	.02
16 oz water	-	16.0	-	-	-	-	-	-	-	-	-	-	-	-
1 box Grainfield's mini cereal	110	-	.5	-	0	-	2.0	24.0	.0	2.00	20.0	.00	-	.04
1 pkt Sweet & Low	2	-	-	.0	0	1	T	T	2.0	-	1.0	-	-	-
1 sl American cheese	210	-	20.0	4.0	45	50	6.1	45.0	5.0	.00	42.0	1.15	1.00	.35
1 carrot	40	-	-	.0	0	-	T	25.0	.0	-	42.0	-	-	-
1 big bagel	185	-	4.8	-	-	-	24.0	122.0	-	24.00	600.0	8.50	.90	7.20
1 tbsp light cream cheese	60	-	6.6	-	15	-	1.0	3.0	3.1	.00	42.0	10.00	-	.01
1 sl challah	95	-	.6	-	-	45	2.5	20.5	-	-	113.0	4.10	-	.70
2 turkey/hamburg hamburgers	1172	46.7	39.9	1.0	128	56	40.2	18.8	3.0	3.10	900.0	62.00	-	5.80
1/2 c mixed vegs: dried tomatoes, zucchini, carrots, squash, onions	150	-	.0	-	0	-	4.0	9.0	.0	4.00	50.0	4.00	-	2.00
8 oz Crystal Light	6	8.0	-	-	-	-	-	-	.2	-	-	-	-	-
8 oz water	-	8.0	-	-	-	-	-	-	-	-	-	-	-	-
8 oz herbal tea	-	8.0	-	-	-	-	-	1.0	-	-	-	-	-	-
2 pkts Sweet & Low	4	-	-	-	-	1	-	-	4.0	-	-	-	-	-
DAILY TOTALS	2225	94.7	83.9	5.0	188	154	81.8	288.3	21.3	9.34	1966.0	89.75	1.90	16.12

T = trace   H = high   L = low   0 = none   - none   % percent

DAY 21

	Calories 1826 Daily	Fluids	Total Fat 60.90 Daily	Polyunsaturated Fats 20.30 Daily	Cholesterol 300 Daily	Weight Grams	Protein 47.90 Daily	Carbohydrates 264.90 Daily	Saturated Fats 18.27 Daily	Fiber 18.27 Daily	Sodium 1200 Daily	Calcium 1200 Daily	Zinc 13.0 Daily	Iron 10.0 Daily
16 oz herbal tea	-	16.0	-	-	-	-	-	-	-	-	-	-	-	-
2 pkts Sweet & Low	4	-	-	-	-	1	-	-	4.0	-	-	-	-	-
4 raw carrots	160	-	T	.0	0	-	T	100.0	.0	-	168.0	-	-	-
8 oz water	-	8.0	-	-	-	-	-	-	-	-	-	-	-	-
8 graham crackers	480	.3	8.9	-	-	94	8.0	80.9	-	-	550.0	30.0	.88	.14
8 oz water	-	8.0	-	-	-	-	-	-	-	-	-	-	-	-
2 sl American cheese	420	-	40.0	8.0	90	100	12.2	90.0	10.0	.0	84.0	2.3	2.00	.70
1/2 regular bagel	83	-	1.4	-	-	-	6.0	30.9	-	.6	198.0	23.0	.29	1.46
17 potato chips	150	-	10.0	-	0	-	2.0	14.0	-	.0	150.0	.0	-	.02
1/2 c tuna salad	383	129.5	19.0	8.5	27	205	32.9	19.3	3.2	-	824.0	35.0	1.15	2.04
1 large green salad	150	-	-	-	-	-	-	50.0	-	8.0	3.3	-	-	2.00
8 oz Crystal Light	6	8.0	-	-	-	-	-	.4	-	-	-	-	-	-
8 oz decaf tea	-	8.0	-	-	-	-	-	1.0	-	-	-	-	-	-
1 tbsp tofu cream cheese	40	-	8.0	6.0	0	-	1.0	1.0	2.0	-	135.0	-	-	-
DAILY TOTALS	1876	177.8	87.3	22.5	117	400	62.1	387.5	19.2	8.6	2112.3	90.3	4.32	6.36

T = trace   H = high   L = low   0 = none   - none   % percent

DAY 22

	Calories 1826 Daily	Fluids	Total Fat 60.90 Daily	Polyunsaturated Fats 20.30 Daily	Cholesterol 300 Daily	Weight Grams	Protein 47.90 Daily	Carbohydrates 264.90 Daily	Saturated Fats 18.27 Daily	Fiber 18.27 Daily	Sodium 1200 Daily	Calcium 1200 Daily	Zinc 13.0 Daily	Iron 10.0 Daily
2 Ry Krisps	70	-	.0	.0	0	-	2.0	14.0	.0	1.0	110.0	.0	-	4.00
2 tbsp tofu cream cheese	80	-	8.0	6.00	0	-	1.0	1.0	2.0	-	135.0	-	-	-
3 graham crackers	260	.1	3.3	-	-	45	4.0	40.2	-	-	325.0	2.0	.42	.75
4 carrots	160	-	T	.00	0	-	T	100.0	.0	-	168.0	-	-	-
1/2 c egg salad	2258	-	15.0	.00	375	-	20.0	2.0	1.1	.0	29.0	10.0	.50	.36
1 little roll	58	-	1.0	-	8	32	2.0	14.0	-	-	80.0	-	-	-
16 oz water	-	16.0	-	-	-	-	-	-	-	-	-	-	-	-
8 oz decaf coffee	2	8.0	T	.00	0	-	T	T	.0	-	1.0	-	-	-
2 pkts Sweet & Low	4	-	-	-	-	1	-	-	4.0	-	-	-	-	-
1 tbsp Intl creamer	35	-	1.5	-	0	-	.0	6.0	-	.0	5.0	.0	-	.00
10 vegetable crackers	150	-	-	-	0	-	2.0	19.0	1.0	1.0	290.0	2.0	-	6.00
2 tbsp tofu cream cheese	80	-	8.0	6.00	0	-	1.0	1.0	2.0	-	135.0	-	-	-
8 oz water	-	8.0	-	-	-	-	-	-	-	-	-	-	-	-
17 potato chips	150	-	10.0	-	0	-	2.0	14.0	-	.0	150.0	.0	-	.02
1 c baked beans	260	-	.0	-	0	-	12.0	48.0	.0	12.0	1100.0	8.0	-	.16
1 big Kosher hot dog	360	-	32.6	.16	70	114	241.8	2.0	24.18	-	1170.0	22.0	2.48	1.40
16 oz Crystal Light	12	16.0	-	-	-	-	-	-	.4	-	-	-	-	-
DAILY TOTALS	3939	48.1	79.4	12.16	453	192	287.8	260.6	30.28	14.0	2712.0	44.0	3.40	14.67

T = trace   H = high   L = low   0 = none   - none   % percent

DAY 23

	Calories 1826 Daily	Fluids	Total Fat 60.90 Daily	Polyunsaturated Fats 20.30 Daily	Cholesterol 300 Daily	Weight Grams	Protein 47.90 Daily	Carbohydrates 264.90 Daily	Saturated Fats 18.27 Daily	Fiber 18.27 Daily	Sodium 1200 Daily	Calcium 1200 Daily	Zinc 13.0 Daily	Iron 10.0 Daily
8 oz decaf coffee	2	8.0	T	.0	0	-	T	T	.0	-	1.0	-	-	-
2 pkts Sweet & Low	4	-	-	-	-	1.00	-	-	4.0	-	-	-	-	-
1 tbsp Intl creamer	35	-	1.5	-	0	-	.00	6.0	-	.0	5.0	.0	-	.00
2 Ry Krisps	70	-	.0	.0	0	-	2.00	14.0	.0	1.0	110.0	.0	-	4.00
1/2 c yogurt	55	-	.0	.0	3	.00	3.00	12.0	.0	.0	36.0	9.0	.00	.00
1/2 c oyster crackers	66	.6	2.0	-	-	16.00	.14	10.6	.4	-	166.0	4.0	-	.20
1 sl challah	95	-	.6	-	-	45.00	2.50	20.5	-	-	113.0	4.1	-	.70
8 oz apple juice	97	-	.0	.1	0	.82	.00	.0	.0	.0	30.0	.0	.00	.00
1 tbsp hummus	25	-	15.0	-	0	-	2.00	2.0	-	1.0	100.0	.0	-	.10
1sm piece grilled salmon	121	58.2	5.4	2.2	47	85.00	16.90	.0	.8	-	37.0	10.0	-	.68
1-1/2 c mixed vegs: cauliflower, carrots, pea pods, zucchini	150	-	.0	-	0	-	4.00	9.0	.0	4.0	50.0	4.0	-	2.00
1 fatayer (spinach tart) - flour, water, spinach, onion, oil spices	220	-	16.0	-	230	123.00	12.00	6.0	-	-	365.0	-	-	-
8 oz Crystal Light	6	8	-	-	-	-	-	.2	-	-	-	-	-	-
8 oz herbal tea	-	8.0	-	-	-	-	-	1.0	-	-	-	-	-	-
2 pkts Sweet & Low	4	-	-	-	-	1.00	-	-	-	-	4.0	-	-	-
8 oz water	-	8.0	-	-	-	-	-	-	-	-	-	-	-	-
DAILY TOTALS	950	90.8	40.5	2.3	280	271.82	42.54	81.3	5.2	6.0	1017.0	31.1	.00	7.68

T = trace   H = high   L = low   0 = none   - none   % percent

* amount exaggerated

DAY 24

	Calories 1826 Daily	Fluids	Total Fat 60.90 Daily	Polyunsaturated Fats 20.30 Daily	Cholesterol 300 Daily	Weight Grams	Protein 47.90 Daily	Carbohydrates 264.90 Daily	Saturated Fats 18.27 Daily	Fiber 18.27 Daily	Sodium 1200 Daily	Calcium 1200 Daily	Zinc 13.0 Daily	Iron 10.0 Daily
4 oz orange juice	75	4.0	.2	.1	0	128	1.5	12.9	.1	-	1.0	1.4	.60	.25
1 slice pineapple	40	.0	.0	.0	0	0	50.0	50.0	.0	6.0	.0	.0	.00	4.00
1/2 c regular bagel	83	-	1.4	-	-	-	6.0	30.9	-	.6	198.0	23.0	.29	1.46
2 tbsp tofu cream cheese	80	-	8.0	6.0	0	-	1.0	1.0	2.0	-	135.0	-	-	-
8 oz water	-	8.0	-	-	-	-	-	-	-	-	-	-	-	-
1/2 c chicken salad	90	-	4.6	-	16	56	8.4	2.16	-	-	156.0	10.0	-	6.80
8 oz decaf coffee	2	8.0	T	.0	0	-	T	T	.0	-	1.0	-	-	-
2 pkts Sweet & Low	4	-	-	-	-	1	-	-	4.0	-	-	-	-	-
1 tbsp Intl creamer	35	-	1.5	-	0	-	.0	6.0	-	.0	5.0	.0	-	.00
1 hard candy	14	-	.1	-	2	-	-	24.0	-	-	12.0	-	-	-
8 oz herbal tea	-	8.0	-	-	-	-	-	-	-	-	-	-	-	-
2 pkts Sweet & Low	4	-	-	-	-	1	-	-	4.0	-	-	-	-	-
Out for Dinner														
3 c decaf coffee	6	24.0	T	.0	0	-	T	T	.0	-	3.0	-	-	-
6 tbsp milk	75	-	6.1	-	0	-	.0	18.0	-	.0	30.0	.0	-	.00
5 pkts Sweet & Low	12	-	-	-	-	5	-	-	-	-	12.0	-	-	-
1 dinner roll	60	-	1.0	-	10	20	2.0	10.0	-	-	65.0	-	-	-
3 oz chicken stir fry carrots, spinach, tomato sauce	350	-	26.0	-	120	119	25.1	42.0	-	-	710.0	-	-	-
1 c vegetables: red/green peppers, onions, carrots	175	-	.0	-	0	-	7.0	20.0	.0	8.0	60.0	5.0	-	3.00
16 oz water	-	16.0	-	-	-	-	-	-	-	-	-	-	-	-
1 Caesar salad	250	-	-	-	-	-	-	100.0	10.0	-	50.0	-	-	3.00
DAILY TOTALS	1355	68.0	48.9	6.1	148	330	101.0	316.96	20.1	14.6	1438.0	39.4	.89	18.51

T = trace   H = high   L = low   0 = none   - none   % percent

DAY 25

	Calories 1826 Daily	Fluids	Total Fat 60.90 Daily	Polyunsaturated Fats 20.30 Daily	Cholesterol 300 Daily	Weight Grams	Protein 47.90 Daily	Carbohydrates 264.90 Daily	Saturated Fats 18.27 Daily	Fiber 18.27 Daily	Sodium 1200 Daily	Calcium 1200 Daily	Zinc 13.0 Daily	Iron 10.0 Daily
8 oz decaf coffee	2	8.0	T	.0	0	-	T	T	.0	-	1.0	-	-	-
1 tbsp Intl creamer	35	-	1.5	-	0	-	.0	6.0	-	.0	5.0	.0	-	.00
2 pkts Sweet & Low	4	-	-	-	-	1	-	-	4.0	-	-	-	-	-
2 tbsp tofu cream cheese	80	-	8.0	6.0	0	-	1.0	1.0	2.0	-	135.0	-	-	-
12 oz Diet Coke w/caffeine	120	12.0	.0	.0	-	-	.0	39.0	-	-	50.0	-	-	-
1 Teriyaki chicken on a stick	200	-	12.0	-	-	75	12.0	12.0	-	-	400.0	7.0	-	-
10 vegetable crackers	150	-	-	-	0	-	2.0	19.0	1.0	1.0	290.0	2.0	-	6.00
2 tbsp tofu cream cheese	80	-	8.0	6.0	0	-	1.0	1.0	2.0	-	135.0	-	-	-
8 oz herbal tea	-	8.0	-	-	-	-	-	1.0	-	-	-	-	-	-
2 pkts Sweet & Low	4	-	-	-	-	1	-	-	4.0	-	-	-	-	-
16 oz water	-	16.0	-	-	-	-	-	-	-	-	-	-	-	-
DAILY TOTALS	675	44.0	29.5	12.0	0	77	16.0	79.0	13.0	1.0	1016.0	9.0	-	6.00

T = trace   H = high   L = low   0 = none   - none   % percent

DAY 26

	Calories 1826 Daily	Fluids	Total Fat 60.90 Daily	Polyunsaturated Fats 20.30 Daily	Cholesterol 300 Daily	Weight Grams	Protein 47.90 Daily	Carbohydrates 264.90 Daily	Saturated Fats 18.27 Daily	Fiber 18.27 Daily	Sodium 1200 Daily	Calcium 1200 Daily	Zinc 13.0 Daily	Iron 10.0 Daily
1 Ry Krisp	35	-	.0	.0	0	-	1.0	7.0	.0	1.0	55.0	.0	-	2.00
1 tbsp tofu cream cheese	40	-	4.0	3.0	0	-	1.0	1.0	1.0	-	70.0	-	-	-
8 oz decaf coffee	2	8.0	T	.0	0	-	T	T	.0	-	1.0	-	-	-
2 pkts Sweet & Low	4	-	-	-	-	1	-	-	4.0	-	-	-	-	-
1 tbsp Intl creamer	35	-	1.5	-	0	-	.0	6.0	-	.0	5.0	.0	-	.00
4 oz orange juice	75	4.0	.2	.1	0	128	1.5	12.9	.1	-	1.0	1.4	.60	.25
16 oz water	-	16.0	-	-	-	-	-	-	-	-	-	-	-	-
1 c chicken soup w/carrots, chicken, celery	233	8.0	9.6	-	-	97	221.2	5.5	1.3	3.4	802.0	13.0	-	.40
1/2 tongue sandwich	283	56.1	20.7	.8	107	100	22.1	.3	8.9	.0	60.0	7.0	17.00	3.39
1 sl pumpernickel bread	82	11.9	.8	-	-	32	2.9	15.4	-	-	173.0	23.0	.36	.88
1 lrg garden green salad	150		-	-	-	-	-	50.0	-	8.0	3.3	-	-	2.00
1/2 vegetable bagel	83	-	1.4	-	-	-	6.0	30.9	-	.6	198.0	23.0	.29	1.46
1 tbsp tofu cream cheese	40	-	4.0	3.0	0	-	1.0	1.0	1.0	-	70.0	-	-	-
1 knishe	135	-	20.0	2.0	50	-	2.0	3.0	3.0	1.0	125.0	-	-	2.00
1 tbsp tofu cream cheese	40	-	4.0	3.0	0	-	1.0	1.0	1.0	-	70.0	-	-	-
1/2 c tuna salad	383	129.5	19.0	8.5	27	205	32.9	19.3	3.2	-	824.0	35.0	1.15	2.04
8 oz Crystal Light	6	8.0	-	-	-	-	-	-	.2	-	-	-	-	-
8 oz herbal tea	-	8.0	-	-	-	-	-	-	1.0	-	-	-	-	-
2 pkts Sweet & Low	4	-	-	-	-	1	-	-	4.0	-	-	-	-	-
DAILY TOTALS	1630	249.5	85.2	20.4	184	564	292.6	154.3	27.7	14.0	2457.3	102.4	19.40	14.42

T = trace   H = high   L = low   0 = none   - none   % percent

DAY 27

	Calories 1826 Daily	Fluids	Total Fat 60.90 Daily	Polyunsaturated Fats 20.30 Daily	Cholesterol 300 Daily	Weight Grams	Protein 47.90 Daily	Carbohydrates 264.90 Daily	Saturated Fats 18.27 Daily	Fiber 18.27 Daily	Sodium 1200 Daily	Calcium 1200 Daily	Zinc 13.0 Daily	Iron 10.0 Daily
2 pkts Sweet & Low	4	-	-	-	-	1	-	-	4.0	-	-	-	-	-
1 tbsp Intl creamer	35	-	1.5	-	0	-	.0	6.0	-	.0	5.0	.0	-	.00
1 Dunkin jelly donut	245	-	10.0	T	30	-	3.0	37.0	6.8	-	143.0	-	-	-
1 baked potato w/chives	145	-	.2	.1	0	156	3.1	33.6	.0	-	8.0	8.0	.45	.55
1 tbsp LF Italian dressing	25	1.1	4.4	2.2	0	7	.0	.2	1.0	-	40.0	.0	.00	.00
1/2 c corn pops	120	-	.0	-	0	-	1.0	28.0	.0	.0	120.0	-	.10	.10
5 pcs grilled chicken	450	-	18.0	-	-	95	18.0	24.0	-	-	400.0	10.0	.50	.50
2 Chicken teriyaki sticks	400	-	24.0	-	-	150	24.0	24.0	-	-	800.0	14.0	-	-
1/2 c cooked squash	18	-	.3	.1	0	90	.8	3.9	.1	1.0	1.0	24.0	.35	.32
1 lrg green salad w/green pepper, carrots, cucumbers	150	-	-	-	-	-	-	50.0	-	8.0	3.3	-	-	2.0
1/2 c white rice	110	-	.1	-	-	103	2.0	25.3	-	-	350.0	11.0	-	.95
4 oz orange juice	75	4.0	.2	.1	8	128	1.5	12.9	.1	-	1.0	1.4	.60	.27
8 oz water	-	8.0	-	-	-	-	-	-	-	-	-	-	-	-
8 oz herbal tea	-	8.0	-	-	-	1	-	-	-	-	4.0	-	-	-
2 pkts Sweet & Low	4	-	-	-	-	1	-	-	4.0	-	-	-	-	-
8 oz Crystal Light	6	8.0	-	-	-	-	-	.2	-	-	-	-	-	-
8 oz water	-	8.0	-	-	-	-	-	-	-	-	-	-	-	-
DAILY TOTALS	1787	37.1	58.7	2.5	38	732	53.4	245.1	16.0	9.0	1875.3	68.4	2.00	4.69

T = trace   H = high   L = low   0 = none   - none   % percent

DAY 28

	Calories 1826 Daily	Fluids	Total Fat 60.90 Daily	Polyunsaturated Fats 20.30 Daily	Cholesterol 300 Daily	Weight Grams	Protein 47.90 Daily	Carbohydrates 264.90 Daily	Saturated Fats 18.27 Daily	Fiber 18.27 Daily	Sodium 1200 Daily	Calcium 1200 Daily	Zinc 13.0 Daily	Iron 10.0 Daily
1/2 c yogurt	55	-	.0	.0	3	0	3.0	12.0	.0	.0	36.0	4.0	-	.20
1 mini box cereal	110	-	.5	-	0	-	2.0	24.0	-	2.0	20.0	.0	-	.40
24 oz water	-	24.0	-	-	-	-	-	-	-	-	-	-	-	-
1 sl challah	95	-	.6	-	-	45	2.5	20.5	-	-	113.0	4.1	-	.70
3 sm homemade donut holes	245	-	10.0	T	30	-	3.0	37.0	6.8	-	143.0	-	-	-
8 oz herbal tea	-	8.0	-	-	-	-	-	1.0	-	-	-	-	-	-
2 pkts Sweet & Low	4	-	-	-	-	1	-	-	4.0	-	-	-	-	-
1 raw carrot	40	-	T	.0	0	-	T	25.0	.0	-	42.0	-	-	-
3/4 c chicken salad	80	-	3.2	-	15	42	7.2	2.0	-	-	142.0	7.0	-	2.00
1 green salad	150	-	-	-	-	-	-	50.0	-	8.0	3.3	-	-	2.00
1 sugar cookie	44	1.3	1.5	-	-	62	1.0	5.9	.7	-	40.0	6.0	-	.12
8 oz herbal tea	-	8.0	-	-	-	-	-	1.0	-	-	-	-	-	-
1 pkt Sweet & Low	2	-	-	-	-	1	-	-	-	-	2.0	-	-	-
DAILY TOTALS	825	41.3	15.8	.0	48	151	18.7	178.0	11.5	10.0	541.3	21.1	-	5.42

T = trace   H = high   L = low   0 = none   - none   % percent

DAY 29

	Calories 1826 Daily	Fluids	Total Fat 60.90 Daily	Polyunsaturated Fats 20.30 Daily	Cholesterol 300 Daily	Weight Grams	Protein 47.90 Daily	Carbohydrates 264.90 Daily	Saturated Fats 18.27 Daily	Fiber 18.27 Daily	Sodium 1200 Daily	Calcium 1200 Daily	Zinc 13.0 Daily	Iron 10.0 Daily
8 oz water	-	8.0	-	-	-	-	-	-	-	-	-	-	-	-
8 oz decaf coffee	2	8.0	T	.0	0	-	T	T	.0	-	1.0	-	-	-
1 tbsp Intl creamer	35	-	1.5	-	0	-	.0	6.0	-	.00	5.0	.0	-	.00
3 tbsp tofu cream cheese	120	-	12.0	9.0	0	-	3.0	3.0	3.0	-	210.0	-	-	-
1 mini bagels	140	-	.0	-	0	-	6.0	30.0	.0	3.00	320.0	.0	-	.60
1 c yellow turnip	45	-	.0	-	0	-	.0	6.0	.0	3.00	75.0	.2	-	.00
1-1/2 c cooked noodles	320	-	2.0	-	0	-	7.0	65.0	.0	2.00	.0	.0	-	.10
1/2 c tomato sauce	50	10.0	.0	-	-	-	2.0	10.0	-	2.00	300.0	.4	-	.20
4 tbsp light Cool Whip	40	-	2.0	-	0	-	.0	4.0	2.0	.00	10.0	.0	-	.00
4 tbsp Smuckers Butterscotch sauce	260	-	2.0	-	10	-	2.0	60.0	.1	.10	140.0	.4	-	.00
1 lrg apple without skin	102	-	.1	.1	0	138	.6	30.4	.2	4.16	2.0	20.0	.10	.50
6 oz apple juice	111	8.0	.3	.1	0	239	.3	27.6	.0	-	17.0	14.0	.90	.61
8 oz herbal tea	-	8.0	-	-	-	-	-	1.0	-	-	-	-	-	-
1 pkt Sweet & Low	2	-	-	-	-	1	-	-	2.0	-	-	-	-	-
8 oz water	-	8.0	-	-	-	-	-	-	-	-	-	-	-	-
DAILY TOTALS	1227	50.0	19.9	9.2	10	378	20.9	243.0	7.3	14.26	1080.0	35.0	1.00	2.01

T = trace   H = high   L = low   0 = none   - none   % percent

DAY 30

	Calories 1826 Daily	Fluids	Total Fat 60.90 Daily	Polyunsaturated Fats 20.30 Daily	Cholesterol 300 Daily	Weight Grams	Protein 47.90 Daily	Carbohydrates 264.90 Daily	Saturated Fats 18.27 Daily	Fiber 18.27 Daily	Sodium 1200 Daily	Calcium 1200 Daily	Zinc 13.0 Daily	Iron 10.0 Daily
8 oz herbal tea	-	8.0	-	-	-	-	-	1.0	-	-	-	-	-	-
2 pkts Sweet & Low	4	-	-	-	-	1	-	-	4.0	-	-	-	-	-
1 large pear	105	-	.16	.8	0	168	.14	50.2	.0	7.2	1.0	38.0	.40	.83
1 sl challah	95	-	.60	-	-	45	2.50	20.5	-	-	113.0	4.1	-	.70
24 oz water	-	24.0	-	-	-	-	-	-	-	-	-	-	-	-
1 c. french fries	300	19.0	18.30	8.8	0	100	4.00	40.0	4.5	.0	216.0	20.0	3.80	7.60
3/4 c to 1c regular cottage cheese	200	-	8.10	.0	30	0	26.00	8.0	6.0	.0	800.0	.1	-	.00
green salad	150	-	-	-	-	-	-	50.0	-	8.0	3.3	-	-	2.00
1 c fresh pineapple	70	-	-	-	-	-	.00	17.0	-	2.0	.0	-	-	.30
8 oz herbal tea	-	8.0	-	-	-	-	-	1.0	-	-	-	-	-	-
1 pkt Sweet & Low	2	-	-	-	-	1	-	-	-	-	4.0	-	-	-
1/2 c cucumbers	7	-	.10	.0	0	52	.30	1.5	.0	.3	1.0	7.0	.12	.21
DAILY TOTALS	933	59.0	27.26	9.6	30	367	32.94	189.2	14.5	17.5	1138.3	69.2	4.32	11.64

T = trace   H = high   L = low   0 = none   - none   % percent

DAY 31

	Calories 1826 Daily	Fluids	Total Fat 60.90 Daily	Polyunsaturated Fats 20.30 Daily	Cholesterol 300 Daily	Weight Grams	Protein 47.90 Daily	Carbohydrates 264.90 Daily	Saturated Fats 18.27 Daily	Fiber 18.27 Daily	Sodium 1200 Daily	Calcium 1200 Daily	Zinc 13.0 Daily	Iron 10.0 Daily
8 oz decaf coffee	2	8.0	T	.0	0	-	T	T	.0	-	1.0	-	-	-
2 tbsp Intl creamer	70	-	2.1	-	0	-	.0	12.0	-	.0	10.0	.0	-	.00
2 pkts Sweet & Low	4	-	-	-	-	1	-	-	4.0	-	-	-	-	-
2 tbsp tofu cream cheese	80	-	8.0	6.0	0	-	1.0	1.0	2.0	-	135.0	-	-	-
1/2 c tuna fish	383	129.5	19.0	8.5	27	205	32.9	19.3	3.2	-	824.0	35.0	1.15	2.04
1/4 c cole slaw	61	36.4	6.0	.0	18	50	1.4	6.0	.0	.0	120.0	22.0	10.00	2.20
3 turkey slices	157	66.3	3.2	.9	69	100	29.9	.0	1.0	.0	64.0	19.0	2.04	.02
1 sl Pepperidge Farm bread (white)	130	-	2.5	-	0	-	4.0	23.0	1.0	1.0	260.0	.4	-	.61
1 sugar cookie	44	1.3	1.5	-	-	62	1.0	59.0	.7	-	40.0	6.0	-	.12
8 oz decaf coffee	2	8.0	T	.0	0	-	T	T	.0	-	1.0	-	-	-
2 pkts Sweet & Low	4	-	-	-	-	1	-	-	4.0	-	-	-	-	-
2 tbsp Intl creamer	70	-	2.1	-	0	-	.0	12.0	-	.0	10.0	.0	-	.00
8 oz regular tea	-	8.0	-	-	-	-	-	2.0	-	-	-	-	-	-
17 potato chips	150	-	10.0	-	0	-	2.0	14.0	-	.0	150.0	.0	-	.20
1 frozen raspberry chill dessert	110	8.0	.0	.0	0	-	.0	46.0	.0	.0	15.0	.0	-	.00
DAILY TOTALS	1267	265.5	54.4	15.4	114	419	72.2	194.3	15.9	1.0	1630.0	82.4	13.19	5.19

T = trace   H = high   L = low   0 = none   - none   % percent

DAY 32

	Calories 1826 Daily	Fluids	Total Fat 60.90 Daily	Polyunsaturated Fats 20.30 Daily	Cholesterol 300 Daily	Weight Grams	Protein 47.90 Daily	Carbohydrates 264.90 Daily	Saturated Fats 18.27 Daily	Fiber 18.27 Daily	Sodium 1200 Daily	Calcium 1200 Daily	Zinc 13.0 Daily	Iron 10.0 Daily
8 oz water	-	8.0	-	-	-	-	-	-	-	-	-	-	-	-
8 oz decaf coffee	2	8.0	T	.0	.0	-	T	T	.0	-	1.0	-	-	-
2 pkts Sweet & Low	4	-	-	-	-	1.0	-	-	4.0	-	-	-	-	-
1 tbsp Intl creamer	35	-	1.5	-	.0	-	.0	6.0	-	.00	5.0	.0	-	.00
1 large bagel	185	-	4.8	-	-	-	24.0	122.0	-	.24	600.0	8.5	.90	7.20
8 oz water	-	8.0	-	-	-	-	-	2.0	-	-	-	-	-	-
8 oz herbal tea	-	8.0	-	-	-	-	-	-	-	-	-	-	-	-
1 medium apple	85	-	T	.5	.1	13.8	.3	21.1	.1	2.80	1.0	1.0	.05	.25
2- 1/2 c romaine lettuce	50	-	.1	-	.0	-	2.0	8.0	.0	2.00	.0	.4	-	.40
5 slices turkey breast	300	68.5	9.6	.2	90.0	150.0	58.2	.0	4.0	.00	170.0	30.0	6.10	.09
8 oz herbal tea	-	8.0	-	-	-	-	-	2.0	-	-	-	-	-	-
2 pkts Sweet & Low	4	-	-	-	-	1.0	-	-	4.0	-	-	-	-	-
DAILY TOTALS	665	108.5	16.0	.7	90.1	165.8	84.5	161.1	12.1	5.04	777.0	39.9	7.05	7.94

T = trace   H = high   L = low   0 = none   - none   % percent

DAY 33

	Calories 1826 Daily	Fluids	Total Fat 60.90 Daily	Polyunsaturated Fats 20.30 Daily	Cholesterol 300 Daily	Weight Grams	Protein 47.90 Daily	Carbohydrates 264.90 Daily	Saturated Fats 18.27 Daily	Fiber 18.27 Daily	Sodium 1200 Daily	Calcium 1200 Daily	Zinc 13.0 Daily	Iron 10.0 Daily
4 oz orange juice	75	4.0	.2	.1	0	128	1.5	12.90	.1	-	1.0	1.4	.60	.25
1/2 c yogurt	55	-	.0	.0	3	0	3.00	12.00	.0	.0	36.0	9.0	.00	.00
1/2 c bagel	83	-	1.4	-	-	-	6.00	30.90	-	.6	198.0	23.0	.29	1.46
4 raw carrots	160	-	T	.0	0	-	T	100.00	.0	-	168.0	-	-	-
1 bite, potato pancake	100	10.2	3.2	1.0	20	22	1.20	8.20	1.1	-	100.0	9.0	.22	.92
16 oz water	-	16.0	-	-	-	-	-	-	-	-	-	-	-	-
16 oz herbal tea	-	16.0	-	-	-	-	-	2.00	-	-	-	-	-	-
3/4 c chicken salad	80	-	3.2	-	15	4.2	7.20	2.00	-	-	142.0	7.0	-	5.20
3 pkts Sweet & Low	6	-	-	-	-	2.0	-	-	6.0	-	-	-	-	-
1 c fresh pineapple	70	-	.0	-	-	-	.00	17.00	-	2.0	.0	-	-	.30
Out for dinner														
1 large salad	150	-	-	-	-	-	-	50.00	-	8.0	3.3	-	-	2.0
1 teriyaki chicken	200	-	12.0	-	-	75.0	12.00	12.00	-	-	400.0	7.0	-	-
1/2 c cooked carrots	45	-	T	.0	0	-	T	25.00	.0	-	42.0	-	-	-
1/2 boiled egg	27	12.7	1.9	-	93	17.0	2.10	.20	-	-	23.0	10.0	.24	.36
1 tbsp blue cheese dressing	25	1.1	4.4	2.2	0	7.0	.00	.20	1.0	-	40.0	.0	.00	.00
1/2 c spinach quiche	220	-	16.0	-	230	123.0	12.00	6.00	-	-	365.0	-	-	-
1/2 c honeydew	66	-	.6	-	-	200.0	.16	14.14	-	-	24.0	28.0	-	-
1/2 c cantaloupe	26	80.2	.2	-	0	80.0	1.00	6.30	-	.1	7.0	9.0	.13	.15
1/2 c FF yogurt ice cream	118	-	3.5	-	-	100.0	3.50	18.70	-	-	-	-	-	-
1/2 c french fries	150	8.1	9.1	4.4	0	50.0	2.00	20.00	2.2	.0	108.0	10.0	1.90	35.00
1 dinner roll	60	-	1.0	-	10	20.0	2.00	10.00	-	-	65.0	-	-	-
1 tbsp Intl creamer	35	-	1.5	-	0	-	.00	6.00	-	.0	5.0	.0	-	.00
1 c chicken soup w/celery, carrots, chicken	233	8.0	9.6	-	-	97.0	221.20	5.50	1.3	3.4	802.0	13.0	-	.40
DAILY TOTALS	1984	156.3	67.8	7.7	371	925.2	274.86	359.04	11.7	14.1	2529.3	126.4	3.38	46.04

T = trace   H = high   L = low   0 = none   - none   % percent

DAY 34

	Calories 1826 Daily	Fluids	Total Fat 60.90 Daily	Polyunsaturated Fats 20.30 Daily	Cholesterol 300 Daily	Weight Grams	Protein 47.90 Daily	Carbohydrates 264.90 Daily	Saturated Fats 18.27 Daily	Fiber 18.27 Daily	Sodium 1200 Daily	Calcium 1200 Daily	Zinc 13.0 Daily	Iron 10.0 Daily
8 oz decaf coffee	2	8.0	T	.0	0	-	T	T	.0	-	1.0	-	-	-
2 pkts Sweet & Low	4	-	-	-	-	1	-	-	4.0	-	-	-	-	-
2 tbsp Intl creamer	70	-	2.1	-	0	-	.0	12.0	-	.0	10.0	.0	-	.00
16 oz water	-	16.0	-	-	-	-	-	-	-	-	-	-	-	-
8 oz orange juice	150	8.0	.4	.2	0	249	1.1	24.9	.2	-	2.0	2.8	.12	.50
1/4 c pretzels	111	.7	1.0	-	-	28	2.6	22.4	-	-	451.0	7.0	.30	.55
1 banana	105	84.7	.6	.1	0	114	1.2	26.7	.2	1.6	1.0	7.0	.19	.35
3 sl turkey breast	157	66.3	3.2	.9	69	100	2.9	.0	1.0	.0	64.0	19.0	2.04	.02
1 sl black forest bread	75	-	1.0	-	0	-	3.0	15.0	-	1.0	160.0	1.0	-	.50
1/2 c FF yogurt	55	-	.0	.0	3	0	3.0	12.0	.0	.0	3.6	9.0	.00	.00
3/4 c strawberries	240	.0	.0	.0	0	-	.0	102.0	.0	4.0	.0	.4	-	.10
2-1/2 c romaine lettuce	50	-	.1	-	0	-	2.0	8.0	.0	2.0	.0	.4	-	.40
8 oz herbal ta	-	8.0	-	-	-	-	-	2.0	-	-	-	-	-	-
2 pkts Sweet & Low	4	-	-	-	-	1	-	-	4.0	-	-	-	-	-
2 tbsp Cool Whip	25	-	1.5	-	-	-	.0	2.0	1.5	-	.0	-	-	-
3/4 -1 c cottage cheese	200	-	8.1	.0	30	0	26.0	8.0	6.0	.0	800.0	.1	-	.0
8 oz herbal tea	-	8.0	-	-	-	-	-	2.0	-	-	-	-	-	-
1 pkt Sweet & Low	2	-	-	-	-	1	-	-	2.0	-	-	-	-	-
2 sl black forest bread	150	-	1.5	-	0	-	6.0	29.0	-	2.0	320.0	2.0	-	.10
8 oz water	-	8.0	-	-	-	-	-	-	-	-	-	-	-	-
DAILY TOTALS	1365	207.7	18.9	1.2	102	494	47.8	260.0	18.9	10.6	1807.6	48.7	2.65	2.52

T = trace   H = high   L = low   0 = none   - none   % percent

DAY 35

	Calories 1826 Daily	Fluids	Total Fat 60.90 Daily	Polyunsaturated Fats 20.30 Daily	Cholesterol 300 Daily	Weight Grams	Protein 47.90 Daily	Carbohydrates 264.90 Daily	Saturated Fats 18.27 Daily	Fiber 18.27 Daily	Sodium 1200 Daily	Calcium 1200 Daily	Zinc 13.0 Daily	Iron 10.0 Daily
8 oz decaf coffee	2	8.0	T	.0	0	-	T	T	.0	-	1.0	-	-	-
2 pkts Sweet & Low	4	-	-	-	-	1	-	-	-	-	4.0	--	-	-
1 tbsp Intl creamer	35	-	1.5	-	0	-	.0	6.0	-	.00	5.0	.00	-	.00
8 oz water	-	8.0	-	-	-	-	-	-	-	-	-	-	-	-
1 sl black forest bread	75	-	1.0	-	0	-	3.0	15.0	-	1.00	160.0	1.00	-	.50
1/2 c cottage cheese	164	-	2.3	.0	0	226	28.0	6.2	1.5	19.00	918.0	138.00	.80	.32
1 bagel (regular)	163	-	2.8	-	-	-	12.0	61.0	-	.12	300.0	46.00	.50	3.00
1 very small slice yellow cake without frosting	126	20.0	.2	-	-	53	3.2	28.6	-	-	269.0	44.0	.05	.23
1 Oscar Mayer Lunchables without cookie	400	-	29.0	-	70	-	13.0	28.0	11.0	1.00	1170.0	.18	-	.80
8 oz decaf coffee	2	8.0	T	.0	0	-	T	T	.0	-	1.0	-	-	-
2 pkts Sweet & Low	4	-	-	-	-	1	-	-	-	-	4.0	-	-	-
2 tbsp Intl creamer	70	-	2.1	-	0	-	.0	12.0	-	.00	10.0	.00	-	.00
8 oz herbal tea	-	8.0	-	-	-	-	-	2.0	-	-	-	-	-	-
1 pkt Sweet & Low	2	-	-	-	-	1	-	-	-	-	2.0	-	-	-
16 oz water	-	16.0	-	-	-	-	-	-	-	-	-	-	-	-
DAILY TOTALS	1047	68.0	38.5	.0	70	282	59.2 H	158.8	12.5	21.12	2844.0 H	229.18	1.35	4.85

T = trace   H = high   L = low   0 = none   - none   % percent

DAY 36

	Calories 1826 Daily	Fluids	Total Fat 60.90 Daily	Polyunsaturated Fats 20.30 Daily	Cholesterol 300 Daily	Weight Grams	Protein 47.90 Daily	Carbohydrates 264.90 Daily	Saturated Fats 18.27 Daily	Fiber 18.27 Daily	Sodium 1200 Daily	Calcium 1200 Daily	Zinc 13.0 Daily	Iron 10.0 Daily
8 oz orange juice	150	8.00	.40	.2	0	249	1.1	24.90	.20	-	2.0	2.8	.12	.50
8 oz decaf coffee	2	8.00	T	.0	0	-	T	T	.00	-	1.0	-	-	-
2 pkts Sweet & Low	4	-	-	-	-	1	-	-	-	-	4.0	-	-	-
2 tbsp Intl creamer	70	-	2.10	-	0	-	.0	12.00	-	.0	10.0	.0	-	.00
2 sl challah	190	-	.12	-	-	90	4.1	40.10	-	-	226.0	8.2	-	1.40
3 oz hard cheese	310	33.90	24.90	.1	71	74	18.3	.24	15.90	.0	380.0	400.0	.74	.14
16 oz water	-	16.00	-	-	-	-	-	-	-	-	-	-	-	-
8 oz herbal tea	-	8.00	-	-	-	-	-	2.00	-	-	-	-	-	-
2-1/2 c romaine lettuce	50	-	.10	-	0	-	2.0	8.00	.00	2.0	.0	.4	-	.40
2 tbsp onion dip with sour cream	81	128.11	4.11	.0	5	74	.9	1.11	2.12	.0	162.0	36.0	.07	.11
2 pkts Sweet & Low	4	-	-	-	-	1	-	-	-	-	4.0	-	-	-
1/2 bagel	83	-	1.40	-	-	-	6.00	30.90	-	.6	198.0	23.0	.29	1.46
8 oz herbal tea	-	8.00	-	-	-	-	-	2.00	-	-	-	-	-	-
2 pkts Sweet & Low	4	-	-	-	-	1	-	-	-	-	4.0	-	-	-
DAILY TOTALS	948	210.01	33.13	.3	76	490	32.4	121.25	18.22	2.6	991.0	470.4	1.22	4.01

T = trace   H = high   L = low   0 = none   - none   % percent

DAY 37

	Calories 1826 Daily	Fluids	Total Fat 60.90 Daily	Polyunsaturated Fats 20.30 Daily	Cholesterol 300 Daily	Weight Grams	Protein 47.90 Daily	Carbohydrates 264.90 Daily	Saturated Fats 18.27 Daily	Fiber 18.27 Daily	Sodium 1200 Daily	Calcium 1200 Daily	Zinc 13.0 Daily	Iron 10.0 Daily
1 c fresh pineapple	70	-	.0	-	-	-	.0	17.0	-	2.00	.0	-	-	.30
24 oz water	-	24.0	-	-	-	-	-	-	-	-	-	-	-	-
16 oz decaf coffee	4	16.0	T	.0	0	-	T	T	.0	-	2.0	-	-	-
4 pkts Sweet & Low	8	-	-	-	-	2	-	-	-	-	8.0	-	-	-
4 tbsp Intl creamer	140	-	4.2	-	0	-	.0	24.0	-	.00	20.0	.0	-	.00
Holiday Party														
1 sl noodle pudding	195	-	13.0	T	30	-	9.0	10.0	H	-	200.0	20.0	-	.10
8 oz IBC soda	180	8.0	.0	-	-	-	.0	48.0	-	-	55.0	-	-	-
2 cheese sticks	476	-	36.0	-	170	-	30.0	42.0	-	-	1500.0	710.0	-	.10
1/2 sl French toast w/1 tbsp strawberry sauce	150	46.2	3.9	-	-	85	6.4	26.8	-	-	220.0	54.0	.08	1.00
1 potato pancake	495	30.3	12.6	2.5	93	76	4.6	26.4	3.4	-	388.0	21.0	.68	1.21
1 sweet potato pancake	144	70.3	3.4	.2	8	105	.9	29.3	1.4	-	73.0	27.0	.16	1.19
1/2 c mandarin orange gelatin mold w/ice cream	184	54.3	7.3	-	-	93	1.8	28.7	1.8	-	112.0	23.0	-	.60
1 sm tuna sandwich	566	142.3	27.8	-	-	255	28.8	52.0	-	-	1288.0	74.0	1.86	2.63
1 tbsp onion dip w/sour cream	30	-	.5	-	0	-	1.0	5.0	.0	1.00	610.0	.2	-	.20
1 oz fudge	113	2.3	3.5	-	-	28	.8	21.3	1.2	-	54.0	22.0	-	.30
1 c fresh fruit: pineapple, honeydew, cantaloupe	57	2.0	.4	-	-	140	1.4	12.4	-	.05	14.0	12.0	.25	.34
1 c red, yellow, and green pepper blend	160	-	.0	-	0	-	6.0	18.0	.0	6.0	50.0	3.0	-	1.00
16 oz herbal tea	-	16.0	-	-	-	-	-	-	-	-	-	-	-	-
DAILY TOTALS	2972	411.7	112.6	2.7	301	784	90.7	360.9	7.8 +H= 14.8	9.05	4594.0	966.2	3.03	8.97

T = trace   H = high   L = low   0 = none   - none   % percent

DAY 38

	Calories 1826 Daily	Fluids	Total Fat 60.90 Daily	Polyunsaturated Fats 20.30 Daily	Cholesterol 300 Daily	Weight Grams	Protein 47.90 Daily	Carbohydrates 264.90 Daily	Saturated Fats 18.27 Daily	Fiber 18.27 Daily	Sodium 1200 Daily	Calcium 1200 Daily	Zinc 13.0 Daily	Iron 10.0 Daily
24 oz water	-	24.0	-	-	-	-	-	-	-	-	-	-	-	-
8 oz decaf coffee	2	8.0	T	.0	0	-	T	T	.0	-	1.0	-	-	-
2 pkts Sweet & Low	4	-	-	-	-	1	-	-	-	-	4.0	-	-	-
2 tbsp Intl creamer	70	-	2.1	-	0	-	.0	12.0	-	.0	10.0	.0	-	.00
1/2 bagel	83	-	1.4	-	-	-	6.0	30.9	-	.6	198.0	23.0	.29	1.46
1 tbsp tofu cream cheese	40	-	4.0	3.0	0	-	1.0	1.0	1.0	-	70.0	-	-	-
1/2 c pears	52	-	.8	.4	0	84	.7	25.1	.0	4.1	1.0	2.4	.20	.41
2 sl pizza	480	-	18.0	T	60	-	28.0	50.0	T	-	1057.0	2.8	-	-
1 c french fries	300	19.0	18.3	8.8	0	100	4.0	40.0	4.5	.0	216.0	20.0	3.80	7.60
1 lrg green salad	150	-	-	-	-	-	-	50.0	-	8.0	3.3	-	-	2.00
2 tbsp blue cheese dressing	50	2.2	8.8	4.4	0	14	.0	.4	2.0	-	80.0	.0	.00	.00
16 oz water	-	24.0	-	-	-	-	-	-	-	-	-	-	-	-
DAILY TOTALS	1231	77.2	53.4	16.6	60	199	39.7	209.4	7.5	12.7	1640.3	48.2	4.29	11.47

T = trace   H = high   L = low   0 = none   - none   % percent

DAY 39

	Calories 1826 Daily	Fluids	Total Fat 60.90 Daily	Polyunsaturated Fats 20.30 Daily	Cholesterol 300 Daily	Weight Grams	Protein 47.90 Daily	Carbohydrates 264.90 Daily	Saturated Fats 18.27 Daily	Fiber 18.27 Daily	Sodium 1200 Daily	Calcium 1200 Daily	Zinc 13.0 Daily	Iron 10.0 Daily
1 c fresh pineapple, honeydew, cantaloupe	57	2.0	.4	-	-	140	1.4	12.4	-	.05	14.0	12.0	.25	.34
8 oz decaf coffee	2	8.0	T	.0	0	-	T	T	.0	-	1.0	-	-	-
2 pkts Sweet & Low	4	-	-	-	-	1	-	-	-	-	4.0	-	-	-
2 tbsp Intl creamer	70	-	2.1	-	0	-	.0	12.0	-	.00	10.0	.0	-	.00
16 oz decaf coffee	4	16.0	T	.0	0	-	T	T	.0	-	2.0	-	-	-
2 pkts Sweet & Low	4	-	-	-	-	1	-	-	-	-	4.0	-	-	-
2 tbsp Intl creamer	70	-	2.1	-	0	-	.0	12.0	-	.00	10.0	.0	-	.00
1-1/2 servings baked scrod w/crumbs	195	-	18.3	-	35	129	23.1	8.4	-	-	130.0	72.0	-	1.00
1/2 c mashed potatoes w/crumbs	111	80.1	4.4	1.3	2	105	2.0	17.5	1.1	.00	309.0	27.0	.29	.28
1/4 c cooked carrots and string bean mix	20	25.0	.2	.1	0	1.0	2.1	6.3	.0	2.00	101.0	11.0	.21	.23
1 lrg green salad	150	-	-	-	-	-	-	50.0	-	8.00	3.3	-	-	2.00
1 tbsp Italian dressing	25	1.1	4.4	2.2	0	7	.0	.2	1.0	-	40.0	.0	.00	.00
8 oz herbal tea	-	8.0	-	-	-	-	-	2.0	-	-	-	-	-	-
1 pkt Sweet & Low	2	-	-	-	-	1	-	-	-	-	2.0	-	-	-
DAILY TOTALS	714	140.2	31.9	3.6	37	385	28.6	120.8	2.1	10.05	630.3	122.0	.75	3.85

T = trace   H = high   L = low   0 = none   - none   % percent

DAY 40

	Calories 1826 Daily	Fluids	Total Fat 60.90 Daily	Polyunsaturated Fats 20.30 Daily	Cholesterol 300 Daily	Weight Grams	Protein 47.90 Daily	Carbohydrates 264.90 Daily	Saturated Fats 18.27 Daily	Fiber 18.27 Daily	Sodium 1200 Daily	Calcium 1200 Daily	Zinc 13.0 Daily	Iron 10.0 Daily
8 oz decaf coffee	2	8.0	T	.0	0	-	T	T	.0	-	1.0	-	-	-
2 pkts Sweet & Low	4	-	-	-	-	1	-	-	-	-	4.0	-	-	-
2 tbsp Intl creamer	70	-	2.10	-	0	-	.0	12.0	-	.0	10.0	.0	-	.000
1/2 bagel	83	-	1.40	-	-	-	6.0	30.9	-	.6	198.0	23.0	.29	1.460
2 tbsp tofu cream cheese	80	-	4.00	6.0	0	-	2.0	2.0	2.0	-	140.0	-	-	-
1 serving grilled chicken on a roll	688	-	40.00	-	82	230	26.0	56.0	8.0	-	1423.0	79.0	1.15	3.300
1/2 c iceberg lettuce	4	26.8	.00	-	-	28	.2	.6	-	-	2.0	6.0	-	.014
16 oz CF Diet Coke	358	16.0	6.52	.0	0	620	.0	88.8	.0	.0	62.0	-	-	.000
1/4 c Harry & David green fried peas	130	-	3.0	-	0	-	7.0	18.0	1.0	5.0	125.0	.2	-	.100
1/2 c fresh fruit mix: honeydew, cantaloupe, pineapple	80	.6	.00	.0	0	30	90.0	30.0	-	.6	9.0	6.0	.08	.120
1 lrg green salad	150	-	-	-	-	-	-	50.0	-	8.0	3.3	-	-	2.000
1/2 c egg salad	225	-	15.00	.0	375	-	20.0	2.0	1.1	.0	29.0	10.0	.50	.360
1/2 c tuna salad	383	129.5	19.00	8.5	27	205	32.9	19.3	3.2	-	824.0	35.0	1.15	2.04
1/2 c drained/washed canned peaches	70	-	.00	-	0	-	1.0	17.0	.0	1.0	10.0	.0	.00	.000
DAILY TOTALS	2327	180.9	91.02	14.5	484	1114	185.1	326.6	15.3	15.2	2840.3	159.2	3.17	9.394

T = trace   H = high   L = low   0 = none   - none   % percent

DAY 41

	Calories 1826 Daily	Fluids	Total Fat 60.90 Daily	Polyunsaturated Fats 20.30 Daily	Cholesterol 300 Daily	Weight Grams	Protein 47.90 Daily	Carbohydrates 264.90 Daily	Saturated Fats 18.27 Daily	Fiber 18.27 Daily	Sodium 1200 Daily	Calcium 1200 Daily	Zinc 13.0 Daily	Iron 10.0 Daily
16 oz water	-	16.0	-	-	-	-	-	-	-	-	-	-	-	-
8 oz decaf coffee	2	8.0	T	.0	0	-	T	T	.00	-	1.0	-	-	-
2 pkts Sweet & Low	4	-	-	-	-	1	-	-	-	-	4.0	-	-	-
2 tbsp Intl creamer	70	-	2.1	-	0	-	.00	12.00	-	.0	10.0	.0	-	.00
1/4 c Harry & David green fried peas	130	-	3.0	-	0	-	7.00	18.00	1.00	5.0	125.0	.2	-	.10
1 c white rice	220	-	.2	-	-	206	4.00	50.60	-	-	700.0	22.0	-	1.90
approx 1 serving Chicken Cashews at a Chinese restaurant	738	.1	38.6	4.5	0	181	20.12	30.87	4.12	.6	410.0	36.0	2.59	3.03
32 oz water	-	32.0	-	-	-	-	-	-	-	-	-	-	-	-
1 lrg green salad	150	-	-	-	-	-	-	50.00	-	8.0	3.3	-	-	2.00
1 sl noodle pudding	195	-	13.0	T	30	-	9.00	10.00	H	-	200.0	20.0	-	.10
1/2 c fresh fruit cantaloupe, honeydew pineapple	80	.6	.0	.0	0	30	90.0	30.00	-	.6	9.0	6.0	.08	.12
1 serving w milk-egg beaters omelet with 1-1/2 c vegetables	200	-	13.0	L	250	-	12.00	8.00	H	1.0	229.0	2.0	-	.20
16 oz water	-	16.0	-	-	-	-	-	-	-	-	-	-	-	-
DAILY TOTALS	1789	72.7	69.9	4.5	280	418	142.12	209.47	5.12	15.2	1691.3	86.2	2.67	7.45

T = trace   H = high   L = low   0 = none   - none   % percent

DAY 42

	Calories 1826 Daily	Fluids	Total Fat 60.90 Daily	Polyunsaturated Fats 20.30 Daily	Cholesterol 300 Daily	Weight Grams	Protein 47.90 Daily	Carbohydrates 264.90 Daily	Saturated Fats 18.27 Daily	Fiber 18.27 Daily	Sodium 1200 Daily	Calcium 1200 Daily	Zinc 13.0 Daily	Iron 10.0 Daily
8 oz decaf coffee	2	8.0	T	.0	0	-	T	T	.0	-	1.0	-	-	-
2 pkts Sweet & Low	4	-	-	-	-	1	-	-	-	-	4.0	-	-	-
2 tbsp Intl creamer	70	-	2.10	-	0	-	.0	12.0	-	.00	10.0	.0	-	.00
1 pear	104	-	.16	.8	0	168	.14	50.2	.0	8.20	2.0	48.0	.40	.82
16 oz water	-	16.0	-	-	-	-	-	-	-	-	-	-	-	-
1 sl Black Forest bread	75	-	1.00	-	0	-	3.00	15.0	-	1.00	160.0	1.0	-	.50
1/2 c canned, drained peaches	70	-	.00	-	0	-	1.00	17.0	.0	1.00	10.0	.0	.00	.00
3 sl turkey breast	157	66.3	3.20	.9	69	100	2.90	.0	1.0	.00	64.0	19.0	2.04	.02
2-1/2 c romaine lettuce	50	-	.10	-	0	-	2.00	8.0	.0	2.00	.0	.4	-	.40
1/2 c egg beaters omelet w/vegetables	200	-	13.00	L	250	-	12.00	8.0	H	1.00	229.0	2.0	-	.20
16 oz water	-	16.0	-	-	-	-	-	-	-	-	-	-	-	-
8 oz herbal tea	-	8.0	-	-	-	-	-	2.0	-	-	-	-	-	-
1 pkt Sweet & Low	2	-	-	-	-	-	1.00	-	-	-	2.0	-	-	-
1/4 c Harry & David green fried peas	130	-	3.00	-	0	-	7.00	18.0	1.0	5.00	125.0	.2	-	.10
1 tbsp light cream cheese	62	18.3	4.70	.1	16	28	2.90	1.8	2.8	.00	160.0	38.0	.21	.40
1 tbsp tofu cream cheese	35	-	1.05	-	0	-	.00	6.0	-	.00	5.0	.0	-	.00
1 bagel (big)	185	-	4.80	-	-	-	24.00	122.0	-	.24	600.0	8.5	.90	7.20
DAILY TOTALS	1146	132.6	33.11	1.8	335	297	55.94	260.0	4.8	18.44	1372.0	117.1	3.55	9.64

T = trace   H = high   L = low   0 = none   - none   % percent

DAY 43

	Calories 1826 Daily	Fluids	Total Fat 60.90 Daily	Polyunsaturated Fats 20.30 Daily	Cholesterol 300 Daily	Weight Grams	Protein 47.90 Daily	Carbohydrates 264.90 Daily	Saturated Fats 18.27 Daily	Fiber 18.27 Daily	Sodium 1200 Daily	Calcium 1200 Daily	Zinc 13.0 Daily	Iron 10.0 Daily
16 oz water	-	16.0	-	-	-	-	-	-	-	-	-	-	-	-
1/2 c canned peaches drained and washed	70	-	.0	-	0	-	1.0	17.0	.0	1.00	10.	.00	.00	.00
1/2 c canned pears drained and washed	80	-	.0	-	0	-	-	19.0	.0	2.00	10.0	.00	-	.00
3 sl turkey breast	157	66.3	3.2	.9	69	100	2.9	.0	1.0	.00	64.0	19.00	2.04	.020
4 oz orange juice	75	4.0	.2	.1	0	128	1.5	12.9	.1	-	1.0	1.40	.60	.250
1 bagel (big)	185	-	4.8	-	-	-	24.0	122.0	-	.24	600.0	8.50	.90	7.200
2 tbsp tofu cream cheese	80	-	4.0	6.0	0	-	2.0	2.0	2.0	-	140.0	-	-	-
16 oz water	-	16.0	-	-	-	-	-	-	-	-	-	-	-	-
Out to celebrate! 16 oz sparkling soda apple/cranberry	215	-	.0	.0	0	360	.5	30.00	.0	-	1.0	-	-	.070
8 hors d'oeuvres: 4 wrapped hot dogs and 4 peking wraps w/vegetables	494	39.6	24.1	.8	35	298	18.9	60.70	6.9	9.37	1109.0	4.36	-	2.177
24 oz Diet Coke	320	24.0	.0	.0	0	360	.0	8.00	.0	.0	2.0	.00	.00	.000
1 lrg garden salad	150	-	-	-	-	-	-	50.00	-	8.0	3.3	-	-	2.000
1/4 c ziti w/tomato sauce	210	-	6.0	-	25	184	12.4	30.00	-	-	720.0	130.00	-	2.000
3 sl turkey breast	157	66.3	3.2	.9	69	100	2.9	.00	1.0	.0	64.0	19.00	2.04	.020
2 sl London Broil	200	25.0	20.2	.1	58	50	18.0	.00	6.3	.0	35.0	7.00	6.00	1.420
1/2 c pasta/kasha varnishkas (groats)	302	121.9	4.9	-	55	194	10.1	56.16	-	-	353.0	7.00	.90	5.000
16 oz decaf coffee	4	16.0	T	.0	0	-	T	T	.0	-	2.0	-	-	-
2 pkts Sweet & Low	4	-	-	-	-	1	-	-	-	-	4.0	-	-	-
2 tbsp half/half	120	.0	2.1	6.8	18	90	88.3	.18	2.2	.0	18.0	36.00	.24	.030
1 sm sl apple pie	282	60.5	11.1	-	-	118	2.4	43.00	-	-	181.0	11.00	.20	1.060
1 sm sl blueberry pie	286	60.2	12.7	-	-	118	2.8	41.20	3.2	-	316.0	13.00	-	.700
1/4 c chopped liver	57	-	3.7	-	-	28	3.8	1.90	-	-	-	3.00	-	2.600
10 vegetable crackers	150	-	-	-	0	-	2.0	19.00	1.0	1.0	290.0	2.00	-	6.000
2 dinner rolls	116	-	2.0	-	15	56	4.0	28.00	-	-	170.0	-	-	-
DAILY TOTALS	3714	515.8	102.2	15.6	344	2185	197.5	541.04	2237	21.61	4093.3	261.26	12.92	30.547

T = trace   H = high   L = low   0 = none   - none   % percent

DAY 44

	Calories 1826 Daily	Fluids	Total Fat 60.90 Daily	Polyunsaturated Fats 20.30 Daily	Cholesterol 300 Daily	Weight Grams	Protein 47.90 Daily	Carbohydrates 264.90 Daily	Saturated Fats 18.27 Daily	Fiber 18.27 Daily	Sodium 1200 Daily	Calcium 1200 Daily	Zinc 13.0 Daily	Iron 10.0 Daily
8 oz decaf coffee ¹/2 c	2	8.0	T	.0	0	-	T	T	.0	-	1.0	-	-	-
2 pkts Sweet & Low	4	-	-	-	-	1	-	-	-	-	4.0	-	-	-
16 oz water	-	16.0	-	-	-	-	-	-	-	-	-	-	-	-
2 tbsp Intl creamer	70	-	2.1	-	0	-	.0	12.0	-	.00	10.0	.0	-	.00
12 strips of peach Juicy Twists	510	-	.0	-	0	-	-	120.0	.0	-	510.0	-	-	-
4 oz Nova Scotia lox	128	-	2.0	-	52	-	20.0	4.0	2.0	-	1680.0	-	-	-
1 big bagel	185	-	4.8	-	-	-	24.0	122.0	-	.24	600.0	8.5	.90	7.20
2 tbsp tofu cream cheese	80	-	4.0	6.0	0	-	2.0	2.0	2.0	-	140.0	-	-	-
8 oz herbal tea	-	8.0	-	-	-	-	-	2.0	-	-	-	-	-	-
2 pkts Sweet & Low	4	-	-	-	-	1	-	-	-	-	4.0	-	-	-
16 oz water	-	16.0	-	-	-	-	-	-	-	-	-	-	-	-
DAILY TOTALS	983	48	12.9	6.0	52	2	46.0	262.0	4.0	.24	2949.0	8.5	.90	7.20

T = trace   H = high   L = low   0 = none   - none   % percent

DAY 45

	Calories 1826 Daily	Fluids	Total Fat 60.90 Daily	Polyunsaturated Fats 20.30 Daily	Cholesterol 300 Daily	Weight Grams	Protein 47.90 Daily	Carbohydrates 264.90 Daily	Saturated Fats 18.27 Daily	Fiber 18.27 Daily	Sodium 1200 Daily	Calcium 1200 Daily	Zinc 13.0 Daily	Iron 10.0 Daily
1/2 bagel	83	-	1.4	-	-	-	6.0	30.90	-	.6	198.0	23.0	.29	1.46
2 tbsp tofu cream cheese	80	-	4.0	6.0	0	-	2.0	2.00	2.0	-	140.0	-	-	-
16 oz water	-	16.0	-	-	-	-	-	-	-	-	-	-	-	-
2 tbsp Intl creamer	70	-	2.1	-	0	-	.0	12.00	-	.0	10.0	.0	-	.00
8 oz decaf coffee	2	8.0	T	.0	0	-	T	T	.0	-	1.0	-	-	-
2 white vanilla sandwich cookies	150	-	6.0	-	0	-	2.0	23.00	1.5	.1	120.0	.0	.00	.40
1 baked potato	145	117.7	.2	.1	0	156	3.1	33.60	.0	-	8.0	8.0	.45	.55
1 tbsp margarine	100	-	11.0	H	7	-	T	.00	L	.0	138.0	.0	.00	.00
1/4 c Harry & David green fried peas	130	-	3.0	-	0	-	7.0	18.00	1.0	5.0	125.0	.2	-	.10
16 oz hot water	-	16.0	-	-	-	-	-	-	-	-	-	-	-	-
1/2 c chicken salad	90	-	4.6	-	16	56	8.4	2.16	-	-	156.0	10.0	-	6.80
1/2 bagel	83	-	1.4	-	-	-	6.0	30.90	-	.6	198.0	23.0	.29	1.46
8 oz apple cider	16	8.0	.0	-	2	0	.0	4.00	.0	.0	30.0	.0	.00	.10
DAILY TOTALS	949	165.7	33.7	6.1	25	212	34.5	156.56	4.5	6.3	1124.0	64.2	1.03	10.87

T = trace   H = high   L = low   0 = none   - none   % percent

DAY 46

	Calories 1826 Daily	Fluids	Total Fat 60.90 Daily	Polyunsaturated Fats 20.30 Daily	Cholesterol 300 Daily	Weight Grams	Protein 47.90 Daily	Carbohydrates 264.90 Daily	Saturated Fats 18.27 Daily	Fiber 18.27 Daily	Sodium 1200 Daily	Calcium 1200 Daily	Zinc 13.0 Daily	Iron 10.0 Daily
8 oz decaf coffee	2	8.0	T	.00	0	-	T	T	.0	-	1.0	-	-	-
2 pkts Sweet & Low	4	-	-	-	-	1	-	-	-	-	4.0	-	-	-
2 tbsp Intl creamer	70	-	2.1	-	0	-	.00	12.0	-	.00	10.0	.00	-	.00
1 bagel (big)	185	-	4.8	-	-	-	24.00	122.0	-	.24	600.0	8.50	.90	7.20
1 tbsp margarine	100	-	11.0	H	7	-	T	.0	L	.00	138.0	.00	.00	.00
1 c Motts cranberry applesauce	180	-	.0	-	0	-	.00	46.0	.0	1.00	.0	-	-	-
6 sl turkey breast	314	132.6	6.4	.18	138	200	58.18	.0	2.0	.00	128.0	.38	4.08	.04
2-1/2 c romaine lettuce	50	-	.1	-	0	-	2.00	8.0	.0	2.00	.0	.40	-	.40
16 oz water	-	16.0	-	-	-	-	-	-	-	-	-	-	-	-
8 oz herbal tea	-	8.0	-	-	-	-	-	2.0	-	-	-	-	-	-
2 pkts Sweet & Low	4	-	-	-	-	1	-	-	-	-	4.0	-	-	-
1 sl Portuguese bread	70	-	1.0	-	0	-	3.00	14.0	.0	1.0	140.0	-	-	-
8 oz hot water	-	8.0	-	-	-	-	-	-	-	-	-	-	-	-
DAILY TOTALS	979	172.6	25.4	.18	145	202	87.18	204.0	2.0	4.24	1025.0	9.28	4.98	7.64

T = trace   H = high   L = low   0 = none   - none   % percent

DAY 47

	Calories 1826 Daily	Fluids	Total Fat 60.90 Daily	Polyunsaturated Fats 20.30 Daily	Cholesterol 300 Daily	Weight Grams	Protein 47.90 Daily	Carbohydrates 264.90 Daily	Saturated Fats 18.27 Daily	Fiber 18.27 Daily	Sodium 1200 Daily	Calcium 1200 Daily	Zinc 13.0 Daily	Iron 10.0 Daily
16 oz water	-	16.00	-	-	-	-	-	-	-	-	-	-	-	-
8 oz decaf coffee	2	8.00	T	.00	0	-	T	T	.0	-	1.0	-	-	-
2 pkts Sweet & Low	4	-	-	-	-	1	-	-	-	-	4.0	-	-	-
2 tbsp Intl creamer	70	-	2.1	-	0	-	.0	12.0	-	.0	10.0	.0	-	.00
4 oz orange juice	75	4.00	.2	.10	0	128	1.5	12.9	.1	-	1.0	1.4	.60	.25
2 tbsp tofu cream cheese	80	-	4.0	6.0	0	-	2.0	2.0	2.0	-	140.0	-	-	-
8 oz decaf coffee	2	8.00	T	.00	0	-	T	T	.0	-	1.0	-	-	-
11 FF garlic and herb crackers	60	-	.0	-	0	-	2.0	12.0	.0	.0	90.0	-	-	.20
1 banana	105	84.70	.6	.10	0	114	1.2	26.7	.2	1.6	1.0	7.0	.19	.35
2-1/2 c romaine lettuce	50	-	.1	-	0	-	2.0	8.0	.0	2.0	.0	.4	-	.40
8 oz water	-	8.00	-	-	-	-	-	-	-	-	-	-	-	-
1/2 c cranberry applesauce	80	-	.0	-	0	-	.0	20.0	-	1.0	20.0	-	-	-
2 c bean soup with franks	374	414.12	14.0	2.12	24	500	20.0	44.0	4.2	-	2184.0	172.0	2.36	4.68
1 tuna pita pocket w/lettuce and pickles	566	142.30	27.8	-	-	255	28.8	52.0	-	-	1288.0	74.0	1.86	2.63
1 sl fresh pineapple core and all	40	-	.0	.00	0	0	.0	65.0	.0	6.0	.0	.0	.00	3.00
16 oz water	-	16.00	-	-	-	-	-	-	-	-	-	-	-	-
DAILY TOTALS	1506	693.12	48.8	8.32	24	998	55.5	254.6	6.5	10.6	3739.0	254.8	5.01	11.51

T = trace   H = high   L = low   0 = none   - none   % percent

DAY 48

	Calories 1826 Daily	Fluids	Total Fat 60.90 Daily	Polyunsaturated Fats 20.30 Daily	Cholesterol 300 Daily	Weight Grams	Protein 47.90 Daily	Carbohydrates 264.90 Daily	Saturated Fats 18.27 Daily	Fiber 18.27 Daily	Sodium 1200 Daily	Calcium 1200 Daily	Zinc 13.0 Daily	Iron 10.0 Daily
16 oz water	-	16.0	-	-	-	-	-	-	-	-	-	-	-	-
8 oz decaf coffee	2	8.0	T	.0	0	-	T	T	.0	-	1.0	-	-	-
2 pkts Sweet & Low	4	-	-	-	-	1	-	-	-	-	4.0	-	-	-
2 tbsp Intl creamer	70	-	2.1	-	0	-	.0	12.0	-	.00	10.0	.0	-	.00
1 blueberry muffin	112	15.6	3.7	-	-	4	2.9	16.8	1.1	-	253.0	34.0	-	.60
4 raw carrots	160	-	T	.0	0	-	T	100.0	.0	-	168.0	-	-	-
1 lrg apple (no skin)	102	-	.1	.1	0	138	.6	30.4	.2	4.16	2.0	20.0	.10	.50
1 tbsp peanut butter	95	.2	8.2	2.5	-	16	4.6	2.5	1.4	-	3.0	5.0	.47	.29
1 tomato basil bagel	185	-	4.8	-	-	-	24.0	122.0	-	.24	600.0	8.5	.90	7.20
3/4 c cottage cheese	185	-	4.9	.0	0	300	35.0	9.9	2.9	22.00	1000.0	150.0	.90	.62
2 tbsp tofu cream cheese	80	-	4.0	6.0	0		2.0	2.0	2.0	-	140.0	-	-	-
8 oz CF Ginseng sports tea	3	8.0	-	-	-	-	-	2.0	-	-	25.0	-	-	-
1 pk Sweet & Low	2	-	-	-	-	1	-	-	-	-	2.0	-	-	-
1 c fresh pineapple	70	-	.0	-	-	-	.0	17.0	-	2.00	.0	-	-	.30
DAILY TOTALS	1070	47.8	27.8	8.6	0	460	69.1	314.6	7.6	28.40	2208.0	217.5	2.37	9.51

T = trace   H = high   L = low   0 = none   - none   % percent

DAY 49

	Calories 1826 Daily	Fluids	Total Fat 60.90 Daily	Polyunsaturated Fats 20.30 Daily	Cholesterol 300 Daily	Weight Grams	Protein 47.90 Daily	Carbohydrates 264.90 Daily	Saturated Fats 18.27 Daily	Fiber 18.27 Daily	Sodium 1200 Daily	Calcium 1200 Daily	Zinc 13.0 Daily	Iron 10.0 Daily
16 oz water	-	16.0	-	-	-	-	-	-	-	-	-	-	-	-
1/2 c corn pops (no milk)	120	-	.0	.0	0	0	1.0	28.0	.0	.0	120.0	.0	.10	.10
8 oz decaf coffee	2	8.0	T	.0	0	-	T	T	.0	-	1.0	-	-	-
2 pkts Sweet & Low	4	-	-	-	-	1	-	-	-	-	4.0	-	-	-
2 tbsp Intl creamer	70	-	2.1	-	0	-	.0	12.0	-	.0	10.0	.0	-	.00
4 oz orange juice	75	4.0	.2	.1	0	128	1.5	12.9	.1	-	1.0	1.4	.60	.25
1 sm pita bread	106	11.9	.6	-	-	38	4.0	20.6	-	.3	215.0	31.0	.30	.92
8 oz herbal tea	-	8.0	-	-	-	-	-	2.0	-	-	-	-	-	-
2 pkts Sweet & Low	4	-	-	-	-	1	-	-	-	-	4.0	-	-	-
1 box Grainfield Oats (mini box, no milk)	80	-	1.0	-	0	-	2.0	16.0	.0	1.0	20.0	.1	-	.20
1/2 c fresh pineapple	35	-	.0	-	-	-	.0	3.0	.0	3.0	.0	-	-	1.50
1-3/4 c (no yolk) extra wide Manischewitz noodles	210	-	1.0	-	0	-	8.0	40.0	.0	2.0	20.0	.0	-	.10
2 tbsp tofu cream cheese	80	-	4.0	6.0	0	-	2.0	2.0	2.0	-	140.0	-	-	-
8 oz herbal tea	-	8.0	-	-	-	-	-	2.0	-	-	-	-	-	-
2 pkts Sweet & Low	4	-	-	-	-	1	-	-	-	-	4.0	-	-	-
2-1/2 c romaine lettuce	50	-	.1	-	0	-	2.0	8.0	.0	2.0	.0	.4	-	.40
DAILY TOTALS 3.47	840	55.9	9.0	6.1	0	169	20.5	146.5	2.1	8.3	539.0	32.9		1.00

T = trace   H = high   L = low   0 = none   - none   % percent

DAY 50

	Calories 1826 Daily	Fluids	Total Fat 60.90 Daily	Polyunsaturated Fats 20.30 Daily	Cholesterol 300 Daily	Weight Grams	Protein 47.90 Daily	Carbohydrates 264.90 Daily	Saturated Fats 18.27 Daily	Fiber 18.27 Daily	Sodium 1200 Daily	Calcium 1200 Daily	Zinc 13.0 Daily	Iron 10.0 Daily
1 banana	105	84.7	.6	.1	0	114	1.2	26.7	.2	1.6	1.0	7.0	.19	.35
2 tbsp tofu cream cheese	80	-	4.0	6.0	0	-	2.0	2.0	2.0	-	140.0	-	-	-
1 c fresh pineapple	70	-	.0	-	-	-	.0	17.0	-	2.0	.0	-	-	.30
1/2 c popcorn	55	-	1.0	-	0	-	2.0	11.0	.0	-	42.0	-	-	-
8 oz decaf coffee	2	8.0	T	.0	0	-	T	T	.0	-	1.0	-	-	-
2 pkts Sweet & Low	4	-	-	-	-	1	-	-	-	-	4.0	-	-	-
2 tbsp Intl creamer	70	-	2.1	-	0	-	.0	12.0	-	.0	10.0	.0	-	.00
8 oz CF Ginseng Sport hot energy drink	3	8.0	-	-	-	-	-	2.0	-	-	25.0	-	-	-
2 pkts Sweet & Low	4	-	-	-	-	1	-	-	-	-	4.0	-	-	-
2-1/2 c romaine lettuce	50	-	.1	-	0	-	2.0	8.0	.0	2.0	.0	.4	-	.40
2 tbsp tofu cream cheese	80	-	4.0	6.0	0	-	2.0	2.0	2.0	-	140.0	-	-	-
1 serving chicken breast w/spices (from frozen pkg)	150	-	1.0	-	70	-	29.0	6.0	.0	1.0	720.0	.4	-	.40
1 c cooked vegetables sweet potato, carrots, onions, sun-dried tomatoes, zucchini	300	-	.0	-	0	-	8.0	18.0	.0	8.0	100.0	8.0	-	4.00
16 oz water	-	16.0	-	-	-	-	-	-	-	-	-	-	-	-
8 oz herbal tea	-	8.0	-	-	-	-	-	2.0	-	-	-	-	-	-
2 pkts Sweet & Low	4	-	-	-	-	1	-	-	-	-	4.0	-	-	-
DAILY TOTALS	977	124.7	12.8	12.1	70	117	46.2	106.7	4.2	14.6	1191.0	15.8	.19	5.45

T = trace   H = high   L = low   0 = none   - none   % percent

DAY 51

	Calories 1826 Daily	Fluids	Total Fat 60.90 Daily	Polyunsaturated Fats 20.30 Daily	Cholesterol 300 Daily	Weight Grams	Protein 47.90 Daily	Carbohydrates 264.90 Daily	Saturated Fats 18.27 Daily	Fiber 18.27 Daily	Sodium 1200 Daily	Calcium 1200 Daily	Zinc 13.0 Daily	Iron 10.0 Daily
16 oz water	-	16.0	-	-	-	-	-	-	-	-	-	-	-	-
8 oz decaf coffee	2	8.0	T	.0	0	-	T	T	.0	-	1.0	-	-	-
2 pkts Sweet & Low	4	-	-	-	-	1	-	-	-	-	4.0	-	-	-
2 tbsp Intl creamer	70	-	2.10	-	0	-	.00	12.0	-	.0	10.0	.0	-	.00
4 oz orange juice	75	4.0	.20	.1	0	128	1.50	12.9	.1	-	1.0	1.4	.60	.25
11 Herb & Garlic FF crackers	2	8.0	T	.0	0	-	T	T	.0	-	1.0	-	-	-
2 tbsp tofu cream cheese	80	-	4.00	6.0	0	-	2.00	2.0	2.0	-	140.0	-	-	-
2 sl challah	190	-	.12	-	-	9.0	4.10	40.1	-	-	226.0	82.0	-	1.40
10 vegetable crackers	150	-	8.00	-	0	-	2.00	19.0	1.0	1.0	250.0	2.0	-	.16
2 tbsp tofu cream cheese	80	-	4.00	6.0	0	-	2.00	2.0	2.0	-	140.0	-	-	-
1 c pears (canned, drained, washed)	104	-	.16	.8	0	168	.14	50.2	.0	8.2	2.0	4.8	.40	.82
16 oz herbal tea	-	16.0	-	-	-	-	-	4.0	-	-	-	-	-	-
2-1/2 c romaine lettuce	50	-	.10	-	0	-	2.0	8.0	.0	2.0	.0	.4	-	.40
1 chicken breast grilled	120	-	8.00	-	40	88	12.0	8.0	.0	5.0	150.0	9.0	1.00	-
1 c cooked vegetables carrots, squash, sun-dried tomatoes, zucchini, onions, sweet potatoes	300	-	.00	-	0	-	8.0	18.0	.0	8.0	100.0	8.0	-	4.00
2 pkts Sweet & Low	4	-	-	-	-	1	-	-	-	-	4.0	-	-	-
10 vegetable crackers	150	-	8.00	-	0	-	2.00	19.0	1.0	1.0	250.0	2.0	-	.16
2 tbsp tofu cream cheese	80	-	4.00	6.0	0	-	2.00	2.0	2.0	-	140.0	-	-	-
16 oz water	-	16.0	-	-	-	-	-	-	-	-	-	-	-	-
DAILY TOTALS	1461	68.0	38.68	18.9	40	395	37.74	197.2	8.1	25.2	1419.0	109.6	2.00	7.19

T = trace   H = high   L = low   0 = none   - none   % percent

DAY 52

	Calories 1826 Daily	Fluids	Total Fat 60.90 Daily	Polyunsaturated Fats 20.30 Daily	Cholesterol 300 Daily	Weight Grams	Protein 47.90 Daily	Carbohydrates 264.90 Daily	Saturated Fats 18.27 Daily	Fiber 18.27 Daily	Sodium 1200 Daily	Calcium 1200 Daily	Zinc 13.0 Daily	Iron 10.0 Daily
16 oz water	-	16.00	-	-	-	-	-	-	-	-	-	-	-	-
1 bagel (big)	185	-	4.8	-	-	-	24.0	122.00	-	.24	600.0	8.50	.90	7.200
2 tbsp tofu cream cheese	80	-	4.0	6.0	0	-	2.0	2.00	2.0	-	140.0	-	-	-
8 oz decaf coffee	2	8.00	T	.0	0	-	T	T	.0	-	1.0	-	-	-
2 tbsp Intl creamer	70	-	2.1	-	0	-	.0	12.00	-	.00	10.0	.00	-	.000
2 pkts Sweet & Low	4	-	-	-	-	1.0	-	-	-	-	4.0	-	-	-
1 sm pita bread toasted w/cinnamon and sugar	124	11.90	.6	-	-	38.0	8.0	24.60	-	.3	215.0	31.00	.30	.920
16 oz herbal tea	-	16.00	-	-	-	-	-	4.00	-	-	-	-	-	-
2 pkts Sweet & Low	4	-	-	-	-	1.0	-	-	-	-	4.0	-	-	-
1/2 spinach tortilla wrap - chicken cubes, teriyaki sauce w/veg	163	50.14	1.2	.0	0	76.0	7.1	31.17	.0	1.90	1365.0	74.00	.60	1.981
1 banana	105	84.70	.6	.1	0	11.4	1.2	26.70	.2	1.60	1.0	7.00	.19	.350
16 oz water	-	16.00	-	-	-	-	-	-	-	-	-	-	-	-
1 tbsp margarine	75	-	11.0	8.0	0	-	-	-	2.0	-	2.5	-	-	-
2 fried egg whites	20	.00	1.0	.0	0	.0	6.0	1.00	2.0	-	45.0	.00	.00	.000
2 tbsp tofu cream cheese	80	-	4.0	6.0	0	-	2.0	2.00	2.0	-	140.0	-	-	-
5 vegetable crackers	75	-	4.0	-	0	-	2.0	16.00	1.0	1.0	125.0	1.50	-	.500
8 oz LC apple cider	16	8.00	.0	.0	0	.0	.0	4.00	.0	.00	30.0	T	.00	T
1 sl American cheese	210	-	20.0	4.0	45	50.0	6.1	45.00	5.0	.00	42.0	1.15	1.00	.350
8 oz water	-	8.00	-	-	-	-	-	-	-	-	-	-	-	-
DAILY TOTALS	1213	1218.74	53.3	24.1	45	176.4	58.4	290.47	14.2	5.04	2724.5	123.15	2.99	11.301

T = trace   H = high   L = low   0 = none   - none   % percent

DAY 53

	Calories 1826 Daily	Fluids	Total Fat 60.90 Daily	Polyunsaturated Fats 20.30 Daily	Cholesterol 300 Daily	Weight Grams	Protein 47.90 Daily	Carbohydrates 264.90 Daily	Saturated Fats 18.27 Daily	Fiber 18.27 Daily	Sodium 1200 Daily	Calcium 1200 Daily	Zinc 13.0 Daily	Iron 10.0 Daily
16 oz water	-	16.00	-	-	-	-	-	-	-	-	-	-	-	-
8 oz decaf coffee	2	8.00	T	.0	0	-	T	T	.0	-	1.0	-	-	-
2 tbsp Intl creamer	70	-	2.1	-	0	-	.0	12.00	-	.00	10.0	.0	-	.000
1 bagel (regular)	163	-	2.8	-	-	-	12.0	61.00	-	.12	300.0	46.0	.50	3.000
2 tbsp tofu cream cheese	80	-	4.0	6.0	0	-	2.0	2.00	2.0	-	140.0	-	-	-
1/2 c LF yogurt	55	-	.0	.0	3	.0	3.0	12.00	.0	.00	36.0	9.0	.00	.000
1 banana	105	84.70	.6	.1	0	11.4	1.2	26.70	.2	1.60	1.0	7.0	.19	.350
2-1/2 c romaine lettuce	50	-	.1	-	0	-	2.0	8.00	.0	2.00	.0	.0	.4	.400
1/2 c spinach tortilla wrap - chicken cubes, teriyaki sauce w/vegetables	163	50.14	1.2	.0	0	76.0	7.1	31.17	.0	1.90	1365.0	74.0	.60	1.981
8 oz Crystal Light	6	8.00	-	-	-	-	-	.20	-	-	-	-	-	-
16 oz water	-	16.00	-	-	-	-	-	-	-	-	-	-	-	-
DAILY TOTALS	694	182.84	10.8	6.1	3	87.4	27.3	153.07	2.2	5.62	1853.0	136.4	1.29	5.731

T = trace   H = high   L = low   0 = none   - none   % percent

DAY 54

	Calories 1826 Daily	Fluids	Total Fat 60.90 Daily	Polyunsaturated Fats 20.30 Daily	Cholesterol 300 Daily	Weight Grams	Protein 47.90 Daily	Carbohydrates 264.90 Daily	Saturated Fats 18.27 Daily	Fiber 18.27 Daily	Sodium 1200 Daily	Calcium 1200 Daily	Zinc 13.0 Daily	Iron 10.0 Daily
16 oz water	-	16.0	-	-	-	-	-	-	-	-	-	-	-	-
4 oz orange juice	75	4.0	.2	.1	0	128.0	1.5	12.9	.1	-	1.0	1.4	.60	.25
1 box Raisin Bran Grainfield cereal	110	-	.5	-	0	-	3.0	27.0	.0	.59	20.0	.0	-	.60
1 banana	105	84.7	.6	.1	0	11.4	1.2	26.7	.2	1.60	1.0	7.0	.19	.35
8 oz decaf coffee	2	8.0	T	.0	0	-	T	T	.0	-	1.0	-	-	-
2 pkts Sweet & Low	4	-	-	-	-	1.0	-	-	-	-	4.0	-	-	-
2 tbsp Intl creamer	70	-	2.1	-	0	-	.0	12.0	-	.00	10.0	.0	-	.00
2 tbsp tofu cream cheese	80	-	4.0	6.0	0	-	2.0	2.0	2.0	-	140.0	-	-	-
4 pc red licorice	140	-	.4	-	0	-	-	52.0	T	.00	40.0	-	-	-
11 Herb & Garlic crackers	60	-	.0	-	0	-	2.0	12.0	.0	.00	90.0	.0	-	.20
1 banana	105	84.7	.6	.1	0	11.4	1.2	26.7	.2	1.60	1.0	7.0	.19	.35
1 tbsp peanut butter	95	.2	8.2	2.5	-	16.0	4.6	2.5	1.4	-	3.0	5.0	.47	.29
16 oz water	-	16.0	-	-	-	-	-	-	-	-	-	-	-	-
2 raw carrots	8	-	T	.0	0	-	T	50.0	.0	-	84.0	-	-	-
1 serving "Trader Giotto's" frozen manicotti spinach florentine	300	-	8.0	-	0	-	19.0	39.0	1.0	20.00	540.0	.2	-	.30
8 oz hot water	-	8.0	-	-	-	-	-	-	-	-	-	-	-	-
16 oz water	-	16.0	-	-	-	-	-	-	-	-	-	-	-	-
DAILY TOTALS	1154	237.6	24.5	8.8	0	167.8	34.5	262.8	4.9	23.79	935.0	20.6	1.45	2.34

T = trace   H = high   L = low   0 = none   - none   % percent

DAY 55

	Calories 1826 Daily	Fluids	Total Fat 60.90 Daily	Polyunsaturated Fats 20.30 Daily	Cholesterol 300 Daily	Weight Grams	Protein 47.90 Daily	Carbohydrates 264.90 Daily	Saturated Fats 18.27 Daily	Fiber 18.27 Daily	Sodium 1200 Daily	Calcium 1200 Daily	Zinc 13.0 Daily	Iron 10.0 Daily
16 oz water	-	16.0	-	-	-	-	-	-	-	-	-	-	-	-
10 vegetable crackers	150	-	-	-	0	-	2.00	.19	1.0	1.0	290.0	2.0	-	1.00
2 tbsp tofu cream cheese	80	-	4.0	6.0	0	-	2.00	2.00	2.0	-	140.0	-	-	-
8 oz decaf coffee	2	8.0	T	.0	0	-	T	T	.0	-	1.0	-	-	-
2 pkts Sweet & Low	4	-	-	-	-	1.0	-	-	-	-	4.0	-	-	-
2 tbsp Intl creamer	70	-	2.1	-	0	-	.00	12.00	-	.0	10.0	.0	-	.00
1/2 c oyster crackers	66	.6	2.0	-	-	16.0	.14	10.60	.4	-	166.0	4.0	-	.20
3 graham crackers	260	.1	3.3	-	-	45.0	4.00	40.20	-	-	325.0	2.0	.42	.75
1 banana	105	84.7	.6	.1	0	11.4	1.20	26.70	.2	1.6	1.0	7.0	.19	.35
2 tbsp tofu cream cheese	80	-	4.0	6.0	0	-	2.00	2.00	2.0	-	140.0	-	-	-
16 oz water	-	16.0	-	-	-	-	-	-	-	-	-	-	-	-
1/2 c sweet canned peas	70	-	.5	-	0	.0	4.00	11.00	.0	3.0	370.0	.2	-	.60
8 oz water	-	8.0	-	-	-	-	-	-	-	-	-	-	-	-
2 fried eggs whites	20	.0	1.0	.0	0	.0	6.00	.00	.0	-	45.0	.0	.00	.00
1 sl turkey bologna	70	-	5.0	-	25	-	4.00	2.00	1.5	.0	350.0	.4	.00	.20
1 sl white Portuguese bread	140	-	1.0	.0	0	.0	6.00	28.00	.0	1.0	280.0	.0	.00	.00
16 oz water	-	16.0	-	-	-	-	-	-	-	-	-	-	-	-
DAILY TOTALS	1117	149.4	23.5	12.1	25	73.4	31.34	134.69	7.1	6.6	2122.0	15.6	.61	3.1

T = trace   H = high   L = low   0 = none   - none   % percent

DAY 56

	Calories 1826 Daily	Fluids	Total Fat 60.90 Daily	Polyunsaturated Fats 20.30 Daily	Cholesterol 300 Daily	Weight Grams	Protein 47.90 Daily	Carbohydrates 264.90 Daily	Saturated Fats 18.27 Daily	Fiber 18.27 Daily	Sodium 1200 Daily	Calcium 1200 Daily	Zinc 13.0 Daily	Iron 10.0 Daily
16 oz decaf coffee	4	16.0	T	.0	0	-	T	T	.0	-	2.0	-	-	-
2 pkts Sweet & Low	4	-	-	-	-	1	-	-	-	-	4.0	-	-	-
2 tbsp Intl creamer	70	-	2.1	-	0	-	.00	12.0	-	.0	10.0	.0	-	.00
1 mini small cupcake w/frosting	120	5.5	3.2	-	-	25	1.00	15.3	-	-	52.0	15.0	-	.15
2 raw carrots	8	-	T	.0	0	-	T	50.0	.0	-	84.0	-	-	-
2 tbsp peanut butter	190	.4	16.4	4.1	-	32	8.12	4.1	2.8	-	6.0	10.0	.94	.58
16 oz water	-	16.0	-	-	-	-	-	-	-	-	-	-	-	-
1 tunafish sandwich	566	142.3	27.8	-	-	255	28.80	52.0	-	-	1288.0	74.0	1.86	2.63
2-1/2 c romaine lettuce	50	-	.1	-	0	-	2.00	8.0	.0	2.0	.0	.4	-	.40
8 oz hot water	-	8.0	-	-	-	-	-	-	-	-	-	-	-	-
11 herb & garlic crackers	60	-	.0	-	0	-	2.00	12.0	.0	.0	90.0	.0	-	.20
8 oz herbal tea	-	8.0	-	-	-	-	-	2.0	-	-	-	-	-	-
2 pkts Sweet & Low	4	-	-	-	-	1	-	-	-	-	4.0	-	-	-
DAILY TOTALS	1076	196.2	49.6	4.1	0	314	41.92	155.4	2.8	2.0	1540.0	99.4	2.80	3.96

T = trace   H = high   L = low   0 = none   - none   % percent

DAY 57

	Calories 1826 Daily	Fluids	Total Fat 60.90 Daily	Polyunsaturated Fats 20.30 Daily	Cholesterol 300 Daily	Weight Grams	Protein 47.90 Daily	Carbohydrates 264.90 Daily	Saturated Fats 18.27 Daily	Fiber 18.27 Daily	Sodium 1200 Daily	Calcium 1200 Daily	Zinc 13.0 Daily	Iron 10.0 Daily
16 oz water	-	16.0	-	-	-	-	-	-	-	-	-	-	-	-
8 oz decaf coffee	2	8.0	T	.0	0	-	T	T	.0	-	1.0	-	-	-
2 pkts Sweet & Low	4	-	-	-	-	1.0	-	-	-	-	4.0	-	-	-
2 tbsp Intl creamer	70	-	2.1	-	0	-	.0	12.0	-	.00	10.0	.0	-	.00
1/2 c LF yogurt w/fruit	150	-	.0	-	5	-	7.0	43.0	.0	-	110.0	.2	-	.00
2 Rye Krisps	70	-	.0	.0	0	-	2.0	14.0	.0	1.00	110.0	.0	-	4.00
3 2-inch ginger snaps	165	-	10.0	L	10	-	1.0	6.0	L	-	205.0	-	-	-
1/2 lb tongue (deli)	460	-	34.0	L	160	-	34.0	T	H	-	238.0	-	-	2.20
1 bagel (regular)	163	-	2.8	-	-	-	12.0	61.0	-	.12	300.0	46.0	.50	3.00
1 tbsp ketchup	16	-	.1	.0	0	.0	.2	2.4	.0	.00	150.0	2.0	.00	.00
8 oz water	-	8.0	-	-	-	-	-	-	-	-	-	-	-	-
8 oz hot water	-	8.0	-	-	-	-	-	-	-	-	-	-	-	-
2 raw carrots	8	-	T	.0	0	-	T	50.0	.0	-	84.0	-	-	-
3/4 c cottage cheese	185	-	4.9	.0	0	300.0	35.0	9.9	2.9	22.00	1000.0	150.0	.90	.62
1 banana	105	84.7	.6	.1	0	11.4	1.2	26.7	.2	1.60	1.0	7.0	.19	.35
1/2 c fresh pineapple	35	-	.0	-	-	-	.0	3.0	.0	3.00	.0	-	-	1.50
1 LF strawberry rice cake	50	-	.0	-	0	-	1.0	11.0	-	-	.0	-	-	-
8 oz hot water	-	8.0	-	-	-	-	-	-	-	-	-	-	-	-
DAILY TOTALS	1483	132.7	54.5	.1	175	312.4	93.4	239.0	3.1	27.72	2213.0	205.2	1.59	11.67

T = trace   H = high   L = low   0 = none   - none   % percent

DAY 58

	Calories 1826 Daily	Fluids	Total Fat 60.90 Daily	Polyunsaturated Fats 20.30 Daily	Cholesterol 300 Daily	Weight Grams	Protein 47.90 Daily	Carbohydrates 264.90 Daily	Saturated Fats 18.27 Daily	Fiber 18.27 Daily	Sodium 1200 Daily	Calcium 1200 Daily	Zinc 13.0 Daily	Iron 10.0 Daily
16 oz water	-	16.0	-	-	-	-	-	-	-	-	-	-	-	-
8 oz decaf coffee	2	8.0	T	.0	0	-	T	T	.0	-	1.0	-	-	-
2 pkts Sweet & Low	4	-	-	-	-	1	-	-	-	-	4.0	-	-	-
2 tbsp Intl creamer	70	-	2.1	-	0	-	.0	12.0	-	.0	10.0	.0	-	.00
1 LF strawberry rice cake	50	-	.0	-	0	-	1.0	11.0	-	-	.0	-	-	-
1/2 c LF yogurt w/fruit	55	-	.0	.0	3	0	3.0	12.0	.0	.0	36.0	9.0	.00	.00
1/2 bagel (regular)	83	-	1.4	-	-	-	6.0	30.9	-	.6	198.0	23.0	.29	1.46
2 tbsp tofu cream cheese	80	-	4.0	6.0	0	-	2.0	2.0	2.0	-	140.0	-	-	-
8 oz water	-	8.0	-	-	-	-	-	-	-	-	-	-	-	-
8 oz hot water	-	8.0	-	-	-	-	-	-	-	-	-	-	-	-
1 c ziti pasta w/tomato sauce	238	9.3	32.9	.0	0	208	9.6	9.1	.0	.0	289.0	.0	.00	.00
1 lrg garden salad	150	-	-	-	-	-	-	50.0	-	8.0	3.3	-	-	2.00
1/2 c 2-inch diameter meatballs	115	-	8.0	L	54	-	9.0	2.0	H	-	64.0	-	-	-
1/2 c tuna fish	383	129.5	19.0	8.5	27	205	32.9	19.3	3.2	-	824.0	35.0	1.15	2.04
8 oz Crystal Light	6	-	.0	.0	0	-	.0	.1	-	-	.0	.0	.00	.00
8 oz hot water	-	8.0	-	-	-	-	-	-	-	-	-	-	-	-
DAILY TOTALS	1236	186.8	67.4	14.5	84	414	63.5	148.4	5.2	8.6	1569.3	67.0	1.44	5.50

T = trace   H = high   L = low   0 = none   - none   % percent

DAY 59

	Calories 1826 Daily	Fluids	Total Fat 60.90 Daily	Polyunsaturated Fats 20.30 Daily	Cholesterol 300 Daily	Weight Grams	Protein 47.90 Daily	Carbohydrates 264.90 Daily	Saturated Fats 18.27 Daily	Fiber 18.27 Daily	Sodium 1200 Daily	Calcium 1200 Daily	Zinc 13.0 Daily	Iron 10.0 Daily
16 oz water	-	16.0	-	-	-	-	-	-	-	-	-	-	-	-
2 pkts Apple Cinnamon Quaker Oats w/hot water	260	4.0	4.00	-	0	+-	6.00	52.0	.0	6.0	200.0	.3	-	.60
8 oz decaf coffee	2	8.0	T	.0	0	`	T	T	.0	-	1.0	-	-	-
2 pkts Sweet & Low	4	-	-	-	-	1	-	-	-	-	4.0	-	-	-
2 tbsp Intl creamer	70	-	2.10	-	0	-	.00	12.0	-	.0	10.0	.0	-	.00
Out for Dinner 3 oz grilled chicken breast	120	-	8.00	-	40	88	12.00	8.0	.0	5.0	150.0	9.0	1.00	-
1 c grilled vegetables red pepper, zucchini	158	-	.0	-	0	-	6.00	10.0	.0	6.0	59.0	6.0	-	2.50
1 c french fries	300	19.0	18.30	8.8	0	100	4.00	40.0	4.5	.0	216.0	20.0	.38	7.60
1 caesar salad	160	-	.60	-	-	136	1.15	28.2	-	-	636.0	48.0	-	.82
24 oz hot water w/taste of tea	-	24.0	-	-	-	-	-	-	-	-	-	-	-	-
3 pkts Sweet & Low	6	-	-	-	-	2	-	-	-	-	6.0	-	-	-
2 sl rye bread	164	224.8	.16	-	-	64	4.18	30.8	-	-	346.0	46.0	.72	1.76
1 tbsp honey dijon dressing	25	1.1	4.40	2.2	0	7	.00	.2	1.0	-	40.0	.0	.00	.00
8 oz hot water	-	8.0	-	-	-	-	-	-	-	-	-	-	-	-
DAILY TOTALS	1269	304.9	37.56	11.0	40	398	33.33	181.2	5.5	17.0	1659.0	1293.0	2.10	13.28

T = trace   H = high   L = low   0 = none   - none   % percent

DAY 60

	Calories 1826 Daily	Fluids	Total Fat 60.90 Daily	Polyunsaturated Fats 20.30 Daily	Cholesterol 300 Daily	Weight Grams	Protein 47.90 Daily	Carbohydrates 264.90 Daily	Saturated Fats 18.27 Daily	Fiber 18.27 Daily	Sodium 1200 Daily	Calcium 1200 Daily	Zinc 13.0 Daily	Iron 10.0 Daily
16 oz water	-	16.0	-	-	-	-	-	-	-	-	-	-	-	-
8 oz decaf coffee	2	8.0	T	.0	0	-	T	T	.0	-	1.0	-	-	-
2 pkts Sweet & Low	4	-	-	-	-	1.0	-	-	-	-	4.0	-	-	-
2 tbsp Intl creamer	70	-	2.1	-	0	-	.0	12.00	-	.00	10.0	.0	-	.00
1 bagel (regular)	163	-	2.8	-	-	-	12.0	61.00	-	.12	300.0	46.0	.50	3.00
2 tbsp tofu cream cheese	80	-	4.0	6.0	0	-	2.0	2.00	2.0	-	140.0	-	-	-
8 oz energy drink Ginseng sport hot tea	3	8.0	-	-	-	-	-	2.00	-	-	25.0	-	-	-
8 oz hot water	-	8.0	-	-	-	-	-	-	-	-	-	-	-	-
2 raw carrots	8.0	-	T	.0	0	-	T	50.00	.0	-	84.0	-	-	-
2-1/2 c romaine lettuce	50	-	.1	-	0	-	2.0	8.00	.0	2.00	.0	.4	-	.40
1/2 c chicken salad	90	-	4.6	-	16	56.0	8.4	2.16	-	-	156.0	10.0	-	6.80
1 c fresh pineapple	70	-	.0	-	-	-	.0	17.00	-	2.00	.0	-	-	.30
6 peach (real fruit) licorice twisters	260	-	.0	-	0	-	.0	62.00	.0	.00	100.0	.0	-	.00
1 banana	105	84.7	.6	.1	0	11.4	1.2	26.70	.2	1.60	1.0	7.0	.19	.35
8 oz water	-	8.0	-	-	-	-	-	-	-	-	-	-	-	-
DAILY TOTALS	905	132.7	14.2	6.1	16	68.4	25.6	242.86	2.2	5.72	821.0	63.4	.69	10.85

T = trace   H = high   L = low   0 = none   - none   % percent

DAY 61

	Calories 1826 Daily	Fluids	Total Fat 60.90 Daily	Polyunsaturated Fats 20.30 Daily	Cholesterol 300 Daily	Weight Grams	Protein 47.90 Daily	Carbohydrates 264.90 Daily	Saturated Fats 18.27 Daily	Fiber 18.27 Daily	Sodium 1200 Daily	Calcium 1200 Daily	Zinc 13.0 Daily	Iron 10.0 Daily
16 oz water	-	16.0	-	-	-	-	-	-	-	-	-	-	-	-
Out for Breakfast														
4 oz orange juice	75	4.0	.20	.1	0	128.0	1.50	12.90	.10	-	1.0	1.4	.60	.25
8 oz decaf coffee	2	8.0	T	.0	0	-	T	T	.00	-	1.0	-	-	-
2 pkts Sweet & Low	4	-	-	-	-	1.0	-	-	-	-	4.0	-	-	-
2 tbsp Intl creamer	70	-	2.10	-	0	-	.00	12.00	-	.00	10.0	.0	-	.00
1 bagel (regular)	163	-	2.80	-	-	-	12.00	61.00	-	.12	300.0	46.0	.50	3.00
2 tbsp light cream cheese	124	36.6	8.14	.2	32	56.0	4.18	2.16	4.16	.00	320.0	76.0	.42	.80
1 banana	105	84.7	.60	.1	0	11.4	1.20	26.70	.20	1.60	1.0	7.0	.19	.35
1 c LF apple cider	16	8.0	.00	.0	0	.0	.00	4.00	.00	.00	30.0	T	.00	T
1-1/2 c vegetable soup (barley, rice, carrots, peas, spices)	244	420.4	6.14	2.8	0	480.0	6.10	38.00	.12	.00	2020.0	112.0	6.24	3.26
8 oz hot water	-	8.0	-	-	-	-	-	-	-	-	-	-	-	-
18 "Old London" cheddar cracker sandwiches	140	-	8.00	.0	0	-	1.00	18.00	4.10	.00	280.0	.5	-	.20
8 oz water	-	8.0	-	-	-	-	-	-	-	-	-	-	-	-
DAILY TOTALS	943	593.7	27.98	3.2	32	676.4	25.98	174.76	8.68	1.72	2967.0	242.9	7.95	7.86

T = trace   H = high   L = low   0 = none   - none   % percent

Note: Went to a birthday party. Had all intentions of eating pizza, cake, ice cream, and soda. Took a banana with me and didn't have any of it!

DAY 62

	Calories 1826 Daily	Fluids	Total Fat 60.90 Daily	Polyunsaturated Fats 20.30 Daily	Cholesterol 300 Daily	Weight Grams	Protein 47.90 Daily	Carbohydrates 264.90 Daily	Saturated Fats 18.27 Daily	Fiber 18.27 Daily	Sodium 1200 Daily	Calcium 1200 Daily	Zinc 13.0 Daily	Iron 10.0 Daily
16 oz water	-	16.0	-	-	-	-	-	-	-	-	-	-	-	-
2 tbsp tofu cream cheese	80	-	4.0	6.0	0	-	2.0	2.0	2.0	-	140.0	-	-	-
8 oz decaf coffee	2	8.0	T	.0	0	-	T	T	.0	-	1.0	-	-	-
2 tbsp Intl creamer	70	-	2.1	-	0	-	.0	12.0	-	.0	10.0	.0	-	.00
4 oz orange juice	75	4.0	.2	.1	0	128	1.5	12.9	.1	-	1.0	1.4	.60	.25
1 c tunafish w/mayo	800	129.5	29.0	18.5	37	405	65.0	38.6	6.4	-	1600.0	70.0	2.30	4.08
2 raw carrots	8	-	T	.0	0	-	T	50.0	.0	-	84.0	-	-	-
18 "Old London" cheddar cracker sandwiches	140	-	8.0	.0	0	-	1.0	18.0	4.1	.0	280.0	.5	-	.20
8 oz water	-	8.0	-	-	-	-	-	-	-	-	-	-	-	-
8 oz hot water	-	8.0	-	-	-	-	-	-	-	-	-	-	-	-
2 sl American cheese	420	-	40.0	8.0	90	100	12.3	95.0	10.0	.0	85.0	310.0	1.20	.75
1 sl Black Forest bread	75	-	1.0	-	0	-	3.0	15.0	-	1.0	160.0	1.0	-	.50
3 oz chicken stir fry w/red, yellow, green peppers and onions	350	-	26.0	-	120	119	25.1	42.0	-	-	710.0	-	-	-
16 oz hot water	-	16.0	-	-	-	-	-	-	-	-	-	-	-	-
8 oz water	-	8.0	-	-	-	-	-	-	-	-	-	-	-	-
DAILY TOTALS	2020	197.5	110.3	32.6	247	752	109.9	285.5	22.6	1.0	3071.0	382.9	4.10	5.78

T = trace　　H = high　L = low　0 = none　- none　% percent

	Calories 1826 Daily	Fluids	Total Fat 60.90 Daily	Polyunsaturated Fats 20.30 Daily	Cholesterol 300 Daily	Weight Grams	Protein 47.90 Daily	Carbohydrates 264.90 Daily	Saturated Fats 18.27 Daily	Fiber 18.27 Daily	Sodium 1200 Daily	Calcium 1200 Daily	Zinc 13.0 Daily	Iron 10.0 Daily
1/2 c Corn Pop cereal	120	-	.0	-	0	-	1.0	-	.0	.0	120.0	.0	.10	.10
16 oz water	-	16.0	-	-	-	-	-	-	-	-	-	-	-	-
8 oz decaf coffee	2	8.0	T	.0	0	-	T	T	.0	-	1.0	-	-	-
2 tbsp Intl creamer	70	-	2.1	-	0	-	.0	12.0	-	.0	10.0	.0	-	.00
4 raw carrots	18	-	T	.0	0	-	T	50.0	.0	-	84.0	-	-	-
1 sm mini cupcake w/frosting	120	5.5	3.2	-	-	25	1.0	15.3	-	-	52.0	15.0	-	.15
1 sl Black Forest bread	75	-	1.0	-	0	-	3.0	15.0	-	1.0	160.0	1.0	-	.50
3 oz chicken stir fry w/red, yellow, green peppers and onions	350	-	26.0	-	120	119	25.1	42.0	-	-	710.0	-	-	-
8 oz water	-	8.0	-	-	-	-	-	-	-	-	-	-	-	-
8 oz hot water	-	8.0	-	-	-	-	-	-	-	-	-	-	-	-
1 tunafish sandwich	566	142.3	27.8	-	-	255	28.8	52.0	-	-	1288.0	74.0	1.86	2.63
1 c grilled red, green, yellow peppers and onions	158	-	.0	-	0	-	6.0	10.0	.0	6.0	59.0	6.0	-	2.50
8 oz Crystal Light	6	8.0	-	-	-	-	-	.1	-	-	-	-	-	-
1 c purple grapes	58	74.8	.3	.1	0	92	.6	15.8	.1	.0	2.0	13.0	.04	.27
DAILY TOTALS	1543	273.3	60.4	.1	120	491	65.5	212.2	.1	7.0	2486.0	109.0	2.00	6.15

T = trace   H = high   L = low   0 = none   - none   % percent

DAY 64

	Calories 1826 Daily	Fluids	Total Fat 60.90 Daily	Polyunsaturated Fats 20.30 Daily	Cholesterol 300 Daily	Weight Grams	Protein 47.90 Daily	Carbohydrates 264.90 Daily	Saturated Fats 18.27 Daily	Fiber 18.27 Daily	Sodium 1200 Daily	Calcium 1200 Daily	Zinc 13.0 Daily	Iron 10.0 Daily
16 oz water	-	16.0	-	-	-	-	-	-	-	-	-	-	-	-
8 oz decaf coffee	2	8.0	T	.0	0	-	T	T	.0	-	1.0	-	-	-
2 pkts Sweet & Low	4	-	-	-	-	1	-	-	-	-	4.0	-	-	-
2 tbsp Intl creamer	70	-	2.1	-	0	-	.0	12.00	-	.0	10.0	.0	-	.00
1 LF strawberry rice cake	50	-	.0	-	0	-	1.0	11.00	-	-	.0	-	-	-
4 oz orange juice	75	4.0	.2	.1	0	128	1.5	12.90	.1	-	1.0	1.4	.60	.25
3 2-inch diameter ginger snap cookies	165	-	10.0	L	10	-	1.0	6.00	L	-	205.0	-	-	-
1/2 c chicken salad	90	-	4.6	-	16	56	8.4	2.16	-	-	156.0	10.0	-	6.80
1 sl Black Forest bread	75	-	1.0	-	0	-	3.0	15.00	-	1.0	160.0	1.0	-	.50
16 oz decaf coffee	4	16.0	-	-	-	-	-	-	-	-	2.0	-	-	-
2 pkts Sweet & Low	4	-	-	-	-	1	-	-	-	-	4.0	-	-	-
2 tbsp Intl creamer	70	-	2.1	-	0	-	.0	12.00	-	.0	10.0	.0	-	.00
3 fig cookies	225	-	4.0	-	0	-	2.0	39.00	2.0	.0	270.0	.0	.00	.20
1/2 c tunafish salad	383	129.5	19.0	8.5	27	205	32.9	19.30	3.2	-	824.0	35.0	1.15	2.04
1 c red, yellow, green sweet peppers	158	-	.0	-	0	-	6.0	10.00	.0	6.0	59.0	6.0	-	2.50
1/2 c Boglhosian tomato basil pita bread	100	-	2.0	-	0	-	3.0	18.00	1.0	1.0	200.0	.8	-	.30
8 oz Crystal Light	6	8.0	-	-	-	-	-	.10	-	-	-	-	-	-
8 oz hot water	-	8.0	-	-	-	-	-	-	-	-	-	-	-	-
DAILY TOTALS	1481	189.5	45.0	8.6	53	391	58.8	157.46	6.3	8.0	1906.0	54.2	1.75	12.59

T = trace   H = high   L = low   0 = none   - none   % percent

DAY 65

	Calories 1826 Daily	Fluids	Total Fat 60.90 Daily	Polyunsaturated Fats 20.30 Daily	Cholesterol 300 Daily	Weight Grams	Protein 47.90 Daily	Carbohydrates 264.90 Daily	Saturated Fats 18.27 Daily	Fiber 18.27 Daily	Sodium 1200 Daily	Calcium 1200 Daily	Zinc 13.0 Daily	Iron 10.0 Daily
16 oz water	-	16.0	-	-	-	-	-	-	-	-	-	-	-	-
8 oz decaf coffee	2	8.0	T	.0	0	-	T	T	.00	-	1.0	-	-	-
2 pkts Sweet & Low	4	-	-	-	-	1	-	-	-	-	4.0	-	-	-
2 tbsp Intl creamer	70	-	2.10	-	0	-	.0	12.0	-	.0	10.0	.0	-	.00
2 strawberry LF rice cake	50	-	.00	-	0	-	1.0	11.0	-	-	.0	-	-	-
2 sl challah	190	-	.12	-	-	90	4.1	40.1	-	-	226.0	8.2	-	1.40
2 sl American cheese	420	-	40.00	8.0	90	100	12.3	95.0	10.00	.0	85.0	310.0	1.20	.75
2-1/2 c romaine lettuce	50	-	.10	-	0	-	2.0	8.0	.00	2.0	.0	.4	-	.40
1-1/2 c vegetable soup: barley, rice, peas w/spices	244	420.4	6.14	2.8	0	480	6.1	38.0	.12	.0	2020.0	112.0	6.24	3.26
16 oz hot water	-	16.0	-	-	-	-	-	-	-	-	-	-	-	-
8 oz water	-	8.0	-	-	-	-	-	-	-	-	-	-	-	-
DAILY TOTALS	1030	468.4	48.46	10.8	90	671	25.5	204.1	10.12	2.0	2346.0	430.6	7.44	5.81

T = trace   H = high   L = low   0 = none   - none   % percent

DAY 66

	Calories 1826 Daily	Fluids	Total Fat 60.90 Daily	Polyunsaturated Fats 20.30 Daily	Cholesterol 300 Daily	Weight Grams	Protein 47.90 Daily	Carbohydrates 264.90 Daily	Saturated Fats 18.27 Daily	Fiber 18.27 Daily	Sodium 1200 Daily	Calcium 1200 Daily	Zinc 13.0 Daily	Iron 10.0 Daily
16 oz water	-	16.0	-	-	-	-	-	-	-	-	-	-	-	-
8 oz decaf coffee	2	8.0	T	.0	0	-	T	T	.0	-	1.0	-	-	-
2 pkts Sweet & Low	4	-	-	-	-	1.0	-	-	-	-	4.0	-	-	-
2 tbsp Intl creamer	70	-	2.1	-	0	-	.0	12.0	-	.0	10.0	.00	-	.00
1 strawberry LF rice cake	50	-	.0	-	0	-	1.0	11.0	-	-	.0	-	-	-
2 tbsp FF cream cheese	60	-	.0	-	10	-	8.0	6.0	.0	.0	300.0	.12	-	.00
1/2 c red and yellow sweet peppers	12	46.4	.2	.1	0	50.0	.4	2.7	.0	.6	2.0	3.00	.90	.63
1/2 banana	53	42.5	.3	.1	0	6.3	1.0	23.4	.1	1.1	1.0	4.00	.90	.17
1/2 c pineapple	20	.0	.0	.0	0	.0	25.0	25.0	.0	3.0	330.0	4.00	-	2.00
Out for dinner														
3.5 oz sirloin tips	208	58.6	8.7	.4	89	100.0	30.4	.0	3.6	.0	66.0	11.00	6.20	3.36
1 c white rice	220	-	.2	-	-	206.0	4.0	50.6	-	-	700.0	22.00	-	1.90
1lrg garden salad	150	-	-	-	-	-	-	50.0	-	8.0	3.3	-	-	2.00
1 sm pita bread	106	11.9	.6	-	-	38.0	4.0	20.6	-	.3	215.0	31.00	.30	.92
4 tbsp Intl creamer	140	-	-	.0	0	24.0	-	-	.0	.0	20.0	-	-	.00
24 oz decaf coffee	6	24.0	T	.0	0	-	T	T	.0	-	3.0	-	-	-
2 pkts Sweet & Low	4	-	-	-	-	1.0	-	-	-	-	4.0	-	-	-
1/2 c cooked zucchini/squash	150	-	.0	-	0	-	4.0	9.0	.0	4.0	50.0	4.00	-	2.00
16 oz hot water	-	16.0	-	-	-	-	-	-	-	-	-	-	-	-
DAILY TOTALS	1255	231.4	12.1	.6	99	426.3	77.8	210.3	3.7	17.0	1709.3	79.12	8.30	12.98

T = trace   H = high   L = low   0 = none   - none   % percent

DAY 67

	Calories 1826 Daily	Fluids	Total Fat 60.90 Daily	Polyunsaturated Fats 20.30 Daily	Cholesterol 300 Daily	Weight Grams	Protein 47.90 Daily	Carbohydrates 264.90 Daily	Saturated Fats 18.27 Daily	Fiber 18.27 Daily	Sodium 1200 Daily	Calcium 1200 Daily	Zinc 13.0 Daily	Iron 10.0 Daily
16 oz water	-	16.0	-	-	-	-	-	-	-	-	-	-	-	-
4 oz orange juice	75	4.0	.2	0.1	0	128	1.5	12.9	0.1	-	1.0	1.4	.6	.25
32 oz hot water throughout morning	-	32.0	-	-	-	-	-	-	-	-	-	-	-	-
8 oz fresh pineapple (core and all!)	70	-	.0	-	-	-	.0	6.0	.0	6.0	.0	-	-	1.50
1/2 c red, green, yellow sweet peppers	12	46.4	.2	.1	0	50	.4	2.7	.0	.6	2.0	3.0	.90	.63
2 sl American cheese	420	-	40.0	8.0	90	100	12.3	95.0	10.0	.0	85.0	310.0	1.20	.75
12 oz Diet CF Pepsi	0	12.0	.0	-	-	-	0	.0	-	-	38.0	-	-	-
2 raw carrots	8	-	T	.0	0	-	T	50.0	.0	-	84.0	-	-	-
1/2 c red, green, yellow sweet peppers	12	46.4	.2	.1	0	50	.4	2.7	.0	.6	2.0	3.0	.90	.63
8 oz water	-	8.0	-	-	-	-	-	-	-	-	-	-	-	-
8 oz hot water	-	8.0	-	-	-	-	-	-	-	-	-	-	-	-
DAILY TOTALS	597	172.8	40.6	8.3	90	328	14.6	169.3	10.1	7.2	212.0	317.4	3.6	3.76

T trace   H high   L low   0 none   - none   % percent

DAY 68

	Calories 1826 Daily	Fluids	Total Fat 60.90 Daily	Polyunsaturated Fats 20.30 Daily	Cholesterol 300 Daily	Weight Grams	Protein 47.90 Daily	Carbohydrates 264.90 Daily	Saturated Fats 18.27 Daily	Fiber 18.27 Daily	Sodium 1200 Daily	Calcium 1200 Daily	Zinc 13.0 Daily	Iron 10.0 Daily
16 oz water	-	16.0	-	-	-	-	-	-	-	-	-	-	-	-
4 oz orange juice	75	4.0	.2	.1	0	128.0	1.5	12.9	.1	-	1.0	1.4	.60	.25
3 2-inch diam ginger snap cookies	165	-	10.0	L	10	-	1.0	6.0	L	-	205.0	-	-	-
1 c purple grapes	58	74.8	.3	.1	0	92.0	.6	15.8	.1	.0	2.0	13.0	.04	.27
1/2 c fresh pineapple	20	.0	.0	.0	0	.0	25.0	25.0	.0	3.0	330.0	4.0	-	2.00
8 oz hot water	-	8.0	-	-	-	-	-	-	-	-	-	-	-	-
3 oz grilled scrod	330	-	20.1	-	40	13.1	23.2	10.2	-	-	298.0	88.0	-	1.0
12 strips Juicy Twists	510	-	.0	-	0	-	-	120.0	.0	-	510.0	-	-	-
1 c grilled vegetables sweet peppers, onions, potatoes, carrots	158	-	.0	-	0	-	6.0	10.0	.0	6.0	59.0	6.0	-	2.50
2-1/2 c romaine lettuce	50	-	.1	-	0	-	2.0	8.0	.0	2.0	.0	.4	-	.40
1/2 piece Bochosian tomato basil pita bread	100	-	2.0	-	0	-	3.0	18.0	1.0	1.0	200.0	.8	-	.30
3 fig squares	225	-	4.0	-	0	-	2.0	39.0	2.0	.0	270.0	.0	.00	.20
12 oz CF diet Pepsi	0	12.0	.0	-	-	-	.0	.0	-	-	38.0	-	-	-
8 oz hot water	-	8.0	-	-	-	-	-	-	-	-	-	-	-	-
8 oz water	-	8.0	-	-	-	-	-	-	-	-	-	-	-	-
DAILY TOTALS	1691	130.8	36.7	.2	50	233.1	64.3	264.9	3.2	12.0	1913.0	113.2	.64	6.92

T = trace   H = high   L = low   0 = none   - none   % percent

DAY 69

	Calories 1826 Daily	Fluids	Total Fat 60.90 Daily	Polyunsaturated Fats 20.30 Daily	Cholesterol 300 Daily	Weight Grams	Protein 47.90 Daily	Carbohydrates 264.90 Daily	Saturated Fats 18.27 Daily	Fiber 18.27 Daily	Sodium 1200 Daily	Calcium 1200 Daily	Zinc 13.0 Daily	Iron 10.0 Daily
16 oz water	-	16.0	-	-	-	-	-	-	-	-	-	-	-	-
8 oz decaf coffee	2	8.0	T	.0	0	-	T	T	.0	-	1.0	-	-	-
1 strawberry LF rice cake	50	-	.0	-	0	-	1.0	11.0	-		.0	-	-	-
12 strips Juicy Twists	510	-	.0	-	0	-	-	120.0	.0	-	510.0	-	-	-
1 banana	105	84.7	.6	.1	0	11.4	1.2	26.7	.2	1.6	1.0	7.0	.19	.35
8 oz hot water	-	8.0	-	-	-	-	-	-	-	-	-	-	-	-
2 sl American cheese	420	-	40.0	8.0	90	100.0	12.3	95.0	10.0	.0	85.0	310.0	1.20	.75
1/2 pc Bochosian tomato basil pita bread	100	-	2.0	-	0	-	3.0	18.0	1.0	1.0	200.0	.8	-	.30
12 oz CF diet Pepsi	0	12.0	.0	-	-	-	.0	.0	-	-	38.0	-	-	-
8 oz hot water	-	8.0	-	-	-	-	-	-	-	-	-	-	-	-
2 raw carrots	80	-	T	.0	0	-	T	50.0	.0	-	84.0	-	-	-
2-1/2 c romaine lettuce	50	-	.1	-	0	-	2.0	8.0	.0	2.0	.0	.4	-	.40
1/2 c cucumber	7	-	.1	.0	0	52.0	.3	1.5	.0	.3	1.0	7.0	.12	.21
1 sl Black Forest bread	75	-	1.0	-	0	-	3.0	15.0	-	1.0	160.0	1.0	-	.50
1/2 c tunafish salad	383	129.5	19.0	8.5	27	205.0	32.9	19.3	3.2	-	824.0	35.0	1.15	2.04
8 oz hot water	-	8.0	-	-	-	-	-	-	-	-	-	-	-	-
8 oz water	-	8.0	-	-	-	-	-	-	-	-	-	-	-	-
DAILY TOTALS	1782	282.2	62.8	16.6	117	368.4	55.7	364.5	14.4	5.9	1904.0	361.2	2.66	4.55

T = trace   H = high   L = low   0 = none   - none   % percent

DAY 70

	Calories 1826 Daily	Fluids	Total Fat 60.90 Daily	Polyunsaturated Fats 20.30 Daily	Cholesterol 300 Daily	Weight Grams	Protein 47.90 Daily	Carbohydrates 264.90 Daily	Saturated Fats 18.27 Daily	Fiber 18.27 Daily	Sodium 1200 Daily	Calcium 1200 Daily	Zinc 13.0 Daily	Iron 10.0 Daily
16 oz water	-	16.0	-	-	-	-	-	-	-	-	-	-	-	-
8 oz decaf coffee	2	8.0	T	.0	0	-	T	T	.0	-	1.0	-	-	-
2 pkts Sweet & Low	4	-	-	-	-	1	-	-	-	-	4.0	-	-	-
2 tbsp Intl creamer	70	-	2.1	-	0	-	.00	12.00	-	.0	10.0	.0	-	.00
1 strawberry LF rice cake	50	-	.0	-	0	-	1.00	11.00	-	-	.0	-		-
2 tbsp peanut butter	190	.4	16.4	4.1	-	32	8.12	4.10	2.8	-	6.0	10.0	.94	.58
1 sm box Grainfield raisin bran cereal	110	-	.5	-	0	-	3.00	27.00	.0	.5	20.0	.0	.00	.60
1/2 c cucumber	7	-	.1	.0	0	52	.30	1.50	.0	.3	1.0	7.0	.12	.21
1/2 c pc Bochusian tomato basil pita bread	100	-	2.0	-	0	-	3.00	18.00	1.0	1.0	200.0	.8	-	.30
1/2 c sweet red, yellow, green peppers	12	46.4	.2	.1	0	50	.40	2.70	.0	.6	2.0	3.0	.90	.63
1/2 c chicken salad	90	-	4.6	-	16	56	8.40	2.16	-	-	156.0	10.0	-	6.80
2 raw carrots	8	-	T	.0	0	-	T	50.00	.0	-	84.0	-	-	-
16 oz hot water	-	16.0	-	-	-	-	-	-	-	-	-	-	-	-
2 sl American cheese	420	-	40.0	8.0	90	100	12.30	95.00	10.0	.0	85.0	310.0	1.20	.75
8 oz water	-	8.0	-	-	-	-	-	-	-	-	-	-	-	-
DAILY TOTALS	1063	94.8	65.9	12.2	106	291	36.52	223.46	13.8	2.4	569.0	340.8	3.16	9.87

T = trace   H = high   L = low   0 = none   - none   % percent

DAY 71

	Calories 1826 Daily	Fluids	Total Fat 60.90 Daily	Polyunsaturated Fats 20.30 Daily	Cholesterol 300 Daily	Weight Grams	Protein 47.90 Daily	Carbohydrates 264.90 Daily	Saturated Fats 18.27 Daily	Fiber 18.27 Daily	Sodium 1200 Daily	Calcium 1200 Daily	Zinc 13.0 Daily	Iron 10.0 Daily
16 oz water	-	16.0	-	-	-	-	-	-	-	-	-	-	-	-
4 oz orange juice	75	4.0	.2	.1	0	128	1.5	12.90	.1	-	1.0	1.4	.60	.25
8 oz decaf coffee	2	8.0	T	.0	0	-	T	T	.0	-	1.0	-	-	-
2 pkts Sweet & Low	4	-	-	-	-	1	-	-	-	-	4.0	-	-	-
2 tbsp Intl creamer	70	-	2.1	-	0	-	.0	12.00	-	.00	10.0	.0	-	.00
1 strawberry LF rice cake	50		.0		0	-	1.0	11.00	-	-	.0	-		
8 oz decaf coffee	2	8.0	T	.0	0	-	T	T	.0	-	1.0	-	-	-
2 pkts Sweet & Low	4	-	-	-	-	1	-	-	-	-	4.0	-	-	-
2 tbsp Intl creamer	70	-	2.1	-	0	-	.0	12.00	-	.00	10.0	.0	-	.00
1 bagel (regular)	163	-	2.8	-	-	-	12.0	61.00	-	.12	300.0	46.0	.50	3.00
1/2 c chicken salad	90	-	4.6	-	16	56	8.4	2.16	-	-	156.0	10.0	-	6.80
1/2 scone w/raisins	186	-	5.3	-	15	63	5.0	29.50	-	-	310.0	117.0	-	1.51
2 raw carrots	8	-	T	.0	0	-	T	50.00	.0	-	84.0	-	-	-
3 fig squares	225	-	4.0	-	0	-	2.0	39.00	2.0	.00	270.0	.0	.00	.20
1 c ziti pasta with tomato sauce	238	9.3	32.9	.0	0	208	9.6	9.10	.0	.00	289.0	.0	.00	.00
1/2 c 2-inch diam meatballs	115	-	8.0	L	54	-	9.0	2.00	H	-	64.0	-	-	-
16 oz hot water	-	16.0	-	-	-	-	-	-	-	-	-	-	-	-
8 oz water	-	8.0	-	-	-	-	-	-	-	-	-	-	-	-
DAILY TOTALS	1302	69.3	62.0	.1	85	457	48.5	240.66	2.1	.12	1504.0	174.4	1.10	11.76

T = trace   H = high   L = low   0 = none   - none   % percent

DAY 72

	Calories 1826 Daily	Fluids	Total Fat 60.90 Daily	Polyunsaturated Fats 20.30 Daily	Cholesterol 300 Daily	Weight Grams	Protein 47.90 Daily	Carbohydrates 264.90 Daily	Saturated Fats 18.27 Daily	Fiber 18.27 Daily	Sodium 1200 Daily	Calcium 1200 Daily	Zinc 13.0 Daily	Iron 10.0 Daily
16 oz water	-	16.0	-	-	-	-	-	-	-	-	-	-	-	-
8 oz decaf coffee	2	8.0	T	.0	0	-	T	T	.0	-	1.0	-	-	-
2 pkts Sweet & Low	4	-	-	-	-	1	-	-	-	-	4.0	-	-	-
2 tbsp Intl creamer	70	-	2.1	-	0	-	.0	12.0	-	.0	10.0	.0	-	.00
8 oz hot water	-	8.0	-	-	-	-	-	-	-	-	-	-	-	-
1 strawberry LF rice cake	50	-	.0	-	0	-	1.00	11.0	-	-	.0	-		
4 raw carrots	16	-	T	.0	0	-	T	100.0	.0	-	168.0	-	-	-
2 sl American cheese	420	-	40.0	8.0	90	100.0	12.30	95.0	10.0	.0	85.0	310.0	1.20	.75
1 c vegetable soup	70	-	1.5	-	-	2.1	2.8	12.1	-	-	730.0	21.0	-	1.50
1/2 c egg salad	225	-	15.0	.0	375	-	20.0	2.0	1.1	.0	29.0	10.0	.50	.36
17 potato chips	150	-	10.0	-	0	-	2.0	14.0	-	.0	150.0	.0	-	.20
3/4 c strawberries	42	132.2	.5	.2	0	138.0	.8	10.0	.0	2.6	2.0	20.0	.17	.55
2 tbsp Cool Whip	25	-	1.5	-	-	-	.0	2.0	1.5	-	.0	-	-	-
8 oz hot water	-	8.0	-	-	-	-	-	-	-	-	-	-	-	-
8 oz water	-	8.0	-	-	-	-	-	-	-	-	-	-	-	-
DAILY TOTALS	1074	180.2	70.6	8.2	603	240.1	38.9	258.1	12.6	2.6	1179.0	361.0	1.87	3.36

T = trace   H = high   L = low   0 = none   - none   % percent

DAY 73

	Calories 1826 Daily	Fluids	Total Fat 60.90 Daily	Polyunsaturated Fats 20.30 Daily	Cholesterol 300 Daily	Weight Grams	Protein 47.90 Daily	Carbohydrates 264.90 Daily	Saturated Fats 18.27 Daily	Fiber 18.27 Daily	Sodium 1200 Daily	Calcium 1200 Daily	Zinc 13.0 Daily	Iron 10.0 Daily
16 oz water	-	16.0	-	-	-	-	-	-	-	-	-	-	-	-
8 oz decaf coffee	2	8.0	T	.0	0	-	T	T	.0	-	1.0	-	-	-
2 pkts Sweet & Low	4	-	-	-	-	1	-	-	-	-	4.0	-	-	-
2 tbsp Intl creamer	70	-	2.1	-	0	-	.0	12.0	-	.0	10.0	.00	-	.00
1/2 bagel	83	-	1.4	-	-	-	6.0	30.9	-	.6	198.0	23.00	.29	1.46
2 tbsp tofu cream cheese	80	-	4.0	6.0	0	-	2.0	2.0	2.0	-	140.0	-	-	-
Out for lunch 8 oz decaf coffee	4	16.0	T	.0	0	-	T	T	.0	-	2.0	-	-	-
4 pkts Sweet & Low	8	-	-	-	-	2	-	-	-	-	8.0	-	-	-
2 tbsp Intl creamer	70	-	2.1	-	0	-	.0	12.0	-	.0	10.0	.00	-	.00
1 serving fried (beer battered) flounder	490	-	28.0	.0	0	210	24.1	39.1	.0	.0	750.0	-	-	-
1 c french fries	300	19.0	18.3	8.8	0	100	4.0	40.0	4.5	0	216.0	20.00	.38	.76
1/4 c coleslaw	61	36.4	6.0	.0	18	50	1.4	6.0	.0	.0	120.0	22.00	10.00	-
8 oz water	-	8.0	-	-	-	-	-	-	-	-	-	-	-	-
4 oz orange juice	75	4.0	.2	.1	0	128	1.5	12.9	.1	-	1.0	1.40	.60	.25
8 oz hot water	-	8.0	-	-	-	-	-	-	-	-	-	-	-	-
8 oz water	-	8.0	-	-	-	-	-	-	-	-	-	-	-	-
8 oz hot water	-	8.0	-	-	-	-	-	-	-	-	-	-	-	-
1 scone (plain)	270	-	9.0	-	10	-	-	41.0	-	2.0	610.0	4.00	-	.10
2 tbsp FF cream cheese	60	-	.0	-	10	-	8.0	6.0	.0	.0	300.0	.12	-	.00
DAILY TOTALS	1577	131.4	71.1	14.9	38	491	47.0	201.9	6.6	2.6	2370.0	70.52	11.27	2.57

T = trace   H = high   L = low   0 = none   - none   % percent

	Calories 1826 Daily	Fluids	Total Fat 60.90 Daily	Polyunsaturated Fats 20.30 Daily	Cholesterol 300 Daily	Weight Grams	Protein 47.90 Daily	Carbohydrates 264.90 Daily	Saturated Fats 18.27 Daily	Fiber 18.27 Daily	Sodium 1200 Daily	Calcium 1200 Daily	Zinc 13.0 Daily	Iron 10.0 Daily
16 oz water	-	16.0	-	-	-	-	-	-	-	-	-	-	-	-
8 oz hot sport energy tea (Ginseng) CF	3	8.0	-	-	-	-	-	2.0	-	-	25.0	-	-	-
1 strawberry LF rice cake	50	-	.0	-	0	-	1.00	11.0	-	-	.0	-		-
4 oz orange juice	75	4.0	.2	.1	0	128	1.5	12.9	.1	-	1.0	1.4	.60	.25
8 oz hot sport energy tea (Ginseng) CF	3	8.0	-	-	-	-	-	2.0	-	-	25.0	-	-	-
3 pkts Sweet & Low	6	-	-	-	-	3	-	-	-	-	6.0	-	-	-
1 sm baked potato	145	117.7	.2	.1	0	156	3.1	33.6	.0	-	8.0	8.0	.45	.55
1/2 c red sweet peppers	12	46.4	.2	.1	0	50	.4	2.7	.0	.6	2.0	3.0	.90	.63
1 c fresh pineapple	70	-	.0	-	-	-	.0	17.0	-	2.0	.0	-	-	.30
2 fried egg whites (in Pam)	20	.0	1.0	.0	0	0	6.0	.0	.0	-	45.0	.0	.00	.00
9 LF wheat thins	120	-	-	.0	0	-	.2	21.0	.5	.2	220.0	.2	-	.40
1 tbsp hummus	25	-	15.0	-	0	-	2.0	2.0	-	1.0	100.0	.0	-	.10
8 oz water	-	8.0	-	-	-	-	-	-	-	-	-	-	-	-
8 oz hot water	-	8.0	-	-	-	-	-	-	-	-	-	-	-	-
DAILY TOTALS	529	216.1	16.6	.3	0	337	14.2	104.12	.6	3.8	432.0	12.6	1.95	2.23

T = trace   H = high   L = low   0 = none   - none   % percent

DAY 75

	Calories 1826 Daily	Fluids	Total Fat 60.90 Daily	Polyunsaturated Fats 20.30 Daily	Cholesterol 300 Daily	Weight Grams	Protein 47.90 Daily	Carbohydrates 264.90 Daily	Saturated Fats 18.27 Daily	Fiber 18.27 Daily	Sodium 1200 Daily	Calcium 1200 Daily	Zinc 13.0 Daily	Iron 10.0 Daily
16 oz water	-	16.0	-	-	-	-	-	-	-	-	-	-	-	-
1/2 bagel (regular)	83	-	1.4	-	-	-	6.00	30.9	-	.6	198.0	23.0	.29	1.46
2 tbsp tofu cream cheese	80	-	4.0	6.00	0	-	2.00	2.0	2.00	-	140.0	-	-	-
8 oz decaf coffee	2	8.0	T	.00	0	-	T	T	.00	-	1.0	-	-	-
2 pkts Sweet & Low	4	-	-	-	-	1	-	-	-	-	4.0	-	-	-
2 tbsp Intl creamer	70	-	2.1	-	0	-	.00	12.0	-	.0	10.0	.0	-	.00
1 strawberry LF rice cake	50	-	.0	-	0	-	1.00	11.0	-	-	.0	-	-	-
1/2 c fresh pineapple	35	-	.0	-	-	-	.00	9.0	-	1.0	.0	-	-	1.50
9 LF wheat crackers	120	-	-	.00	0	-	.20	21.0	.50	.2	220.0	.2	-	.40
1/2 c tunafish salad	383	129.5	19.0	8.50	27	205	32.90	19.3	3.20	-	824.0	35.0	1.15	2.04
8 o water	-	8.0	-	-	-	-	-	-	-	-	-	-	-	-
1/4 c pitted dates	130	-	.0	-	-	-	1.00	31.0	-	-	.0	-	-	-
3 2-inch diameter gingersnap cookies	165	-	10.0	L	10	-	1.00	6.0	L	-	205.0	-	-	-
1 lrg kosher hot dog	360	-	32.6	.16	70	114	24.18	2.0	24.18	-	1170.0	22.0	2.48	1.40
1 c vegetarian baked beans	260	-	.0	-	0	-	12.00	48.0	.00	12.0	1100.0	8.0	-	.16
4 sl mandarin orange	111	-	.1	.00	0	140	1.40	16.3	.00	.0	1.0	56.0	.08	.17
8 oz hot water	-	8.0	-	-	-	-	-	-	-	-	-	-	-	-
1 sl black forest bread	75	-	1.0	-	0	-	3.00	15.0	-	1.0	160.0	-	-	.50
8 oz water	-	8.0	-	-	-	-	-	-	-	-	-	-	-	-
DAILY TOTALS	1928	177.5	70.2	14.66	107	460	84.68	223.5	29.88	14.8	4033.0	144.2	4.00	6.28

T = trace   H = high   L = low   0 = none   - none   % percent

DAY 76

	Calories 1826 Daily	Fluids	Total Fat 60.90 Daily	Polyunsaturated Fats 20.30 Daily	Cholesterol 300 Daily	Weight Grams	Protein 47.90 Daily	Carbohydrates 264.90 Daily	Saturated Fats 18.27 Daily	Fiber 18.27 Daily	Sodium 1200 Daily	Calcium 1200 Daily	Zinc 13.0 Daily	Iron 10.0 Daily
16 oz water	-	16.0	-	-	-	-	-	-	-	-	-	-	-	-
8 oz decaf coffee	2	8.0	T	.0	0	-	T	T	.0	-	1.0	-	-	-
2 pkts Sweet & Low	4	-	-	-	-	1.0	-	-	-	-	4.0	-	-	-
2 tbsp Intl creamer	70	-	2.1	-	0	-	.0	12.0	-	.0	10.0	.0	-	.00
1 strawberry LF rice cake	50	-	.0	-	0	-	1.0	11.0	-	-	.0	-	-	-
2 tbsp tofu cream cheese	80	-	4.0	6.0	0	-	2.0	2.0	2.0	-	140.0	-	-	-
1 c Healthy Valley FF vegetable soup in a cup	110	-	.0	-	0	-	5.0	24.0	.0	3.0	190.0	.2	-	.80
1 banana	105	84.7	.6	.1	0	11.4	1.2	26.7	.2	1.6	1.0	7.0	.19	.35
1/4 c pitted dates	130	-	.0	-	-	-	1.0	31.0	-	-	.0	-	-	-
1 medium fig	37	39.6	.2	.1	0	50.0	.4	9.6	.0	-	1.0	18.0	.70	.18
3 2-inch diameter gingersnap cookies	165	-	10.0	L	10	-	1.0	6.0	L	-	205.0	-	-	-
8 oz hot water	-	8.0	-	-	-	-	-	-	-	-	-	-	-	-
8 oz water	-	8.0	-	-	-	-	-	-	-	-	-	-	-	-
2-1/2 c romaine lettuce	50	-	.1	-	0	-	2.0	8.0	.0	2.0	.0	.4	-	.40
1/2 c egg salad	225	-	15.0	.0	375	-	20.0	2.0	1.1	.0	29.0	10.0	.50	.36
1/2 sl Bochusian tomato basil pita bread	100	-	2.0	-	0	-	3.0	18.0	1.0	1.0	200.0	.8	-	.30
1/2 c yellow sweet peppers	12	46.4	.2	.1	0	50.0	.4	2.7	.0	.6	2.0	3.0	.90	.63
1/2 c sugar free Jello	8	4.0	.0	-	0	-	1.0	.0	-	-	50.0	-	-	-
1/2 c fresh pineapple	35	-	.0	-	-	-	.0	9.0	-	1.0	.0	-	-	1.50
8 oz hot water	-	8.0	-	-	-	-	-	-	-	-	-	-	-	-
DAILY TOTALS	1183	222.7	34.2	6.3	385	112.4	38.0	162.3	4.3	9.2	833.0	39.4	2.29	4.52

T = trace   H = high   L = low   0 = none   - none   % percent

	Calories 1826 Daily	Fluids	Total Fat 60.90 Daily	Polyunsaturated Fats 20.30 Daily	Cholesterol 300 Daily	Weight Grams	Protein 47.90 Daily	Carbohydrates 264.90 Daily	Saturated Fats 18.27 Daily	Fiber 18.27 Daily	Sodium 1200 Daily	Calcium 1200 Daily	Zinc 13.0 Daily	Iron 10.0 Daily
16 oz water	-	16.0	-	-	-	-	-	-	-	-	-	-		-
1 strawberry LF rice cake	50	-	.0	-	0	-	1.0	11.00	-	-	.0	-		-
8 oz decaf coffee	2	8.0	T	.0	0	-	T	T	.0	-	1.0	-	-	-
2 pkts Sweet & Low	4	-	-	-	-	1.0	-	-	-	-	4.0	-	-	-
2 tbsp Intl creamer	70	-	2.1	-	0	-	.0	12.00	-	.0	10.0	.0	-	.00
1 banana	105	84.7	.6	.1	0	11.4	1.2	26.70	.2	1.6	1.0	7.0	.19	.35
1/2 bagel (regular)	83	-	1.4	-	-	-	6.0	30.90	-	.6	198.0	23.0	.29	1.46
1/2 c fresh pineapple	20	.0	.0	.0	0	.0	25.0	25.00	.0	3.0	330.0	4.0	.90	.63
3 2-inch diameter gingersnap cookies	165	-	10.0	L	10.0	-	1.0	6.00	L	-	205.0	-	-	-
2 raw carrots	8	-	T	.0	0	-	T	50.00	.0	-	84.0	-	-	-
15 pc Richardson jelly candy	110	-	.0	-	-	-	.0	40.00	-	-	10.0	-	-	-
1/2 c chicken salad	90	-	4.6	-	16	56.0	8.4	2.16	-	-	156.0	10.0	-	6.80
8 oz hot water	-	8.0	-	-	-	-	-	-	-	-	-	-	-	-
2-1/2 c romaine lettuce	50	-	.1	-	0	-	2.0	8.00	.0	2.0	.0	.4	-	.40
1 c grilled vegetables peppers, potatoes, carrots, onions	175	-	.0	-	0	-	7.0	20.00	.0	8.0	60.0	5.0	-	3.00
1/2 c SF Jello	8	4.0	.0	-	0	-	1.0	.00	-	-	50.0	-	-	-
2 tbsp Cool Whip	25	-	1.5	-	-	-	.0	2.00	1.5	-	.0	-	-	-
8 oz hot water	-	8.0	-	-	-	-	-	-	-	-	-	-	-	-
8 oz water	-	8.0	-	-	-	-	-	-	-	-	-	-	-	-
DAILY TOTALS	965	136.7	20.3	.1	26	68.4	52.6	233.76	1.7	15.2	1109.0	49.4	1.38	12.64

T = trace   H = high   L = low   0 = none   - none   % percent

DAY 78

	Calories 1826 Daily	Fluids	Total Fat 60.90 Daily	Polyunsaturated Fats 20.30 Daily	Cholesterol 300 Daily	Weight Grams	Protein 47.90 Daily	Carbohydrates 264.90 Daily	Saturated Fats 18.27 Daily	Fiber 18.27 Daily	Sodium 1200 Daily	Calcium 1200 Daily	Zinc 13.0 Daily	Iron 10.0 Daily
16 oz water	-	16.0	-	-	-	-	-	-	-	-	-	-	-	-
8 oz decaf coffee	2	8.0	T	.0	0	-	T	T	.0	-	1.0	-	-	-
2 pkts Sweet & Low	4	-	-	-	-	1.000	-	-	-	-	4.0	-	-	-
2 tbsp Intl creamer	70	-	2.1	-	0	-	.0	12.00	-	.00	10.0	.0	-	.00
1 blueberry muffin	112	15.6	3.7	-	-	4.000	2.9	16.80	1.1	-	253.0	34.0	-	.60
1/4 c pretzels	111	.7	1.0	-	-	28.000	2.6	22.40	-	-	451.0	7.0	.30	.55
8 oz apple juice	194	-	.0	.2	0	.164	.0	.00	.0	.00	60.0	.0	.00	.00
1 bagel (regular)	166	-	2.8	-	-	-	12.0	60.18	-	.12	396.0	46.0	.58	1.26
2 tbsp tofu cream cheese	80	-	4.0	6.0	0	-	2.0	2.00	2.0	-	140.0	-	-	-
2-1/2 c romaine lettuce	50	-	.1	-	0	-	2.0	8.00	.0	2.00	.0	.4	-	.40
1/2 c tunafish salad	383	129.5	19.0	8.5	27	205.000	32.9	19.30	3.2	-	824.0	35.0	1.15	2.04
1/2 c sweet red, peppers	12	46.4	.2	.1	0	50.000	.4	2.70	.0	.60	2.0	3.0	.90	.63
8 oz hot water	-	8.0	-	-	-	-	-	-	-	-	-	-	-	-
1 sl angel food cake	140	-	.0	-	0	-	3.0	32.00	.0	.00	350.0	.2	-	.20
8 oz water	-	8.0	-	-	-	-	-	-	-	-	-	-	-	-
DAILY TOTALS	1324	232.2	32.9	14.8	27	288.164	57.8	175.38	6.3	2.72	2491.0	125.6	2.93	5.68

T = trace   H = high   L = low   0 = none   - none   % percent

DAY 79

	Calories 1826 Daily	Fluids	Total Fat 60.90 Daily	Polyunsaturated Fats 20.30 Daily	Cholesterol 300 Daily	Weight Grams	Protein 47.90 Daily	Carbohydrates 264.90 Daily	Saturated Fats 18.27 Daily	Fiber 18.27 Daily	Sodium 1200 Daily	Calcium 1200 Daily	Zinc 13.0 Daily	Iron 10.0 Daily
16 oz water	-	16.0	-	-	-	-	-	-	-	-	-	-	-	-
8 oz decaf coffee	2	8.0	T	.0	0	-	T	T	.0	-	1.0	-	-	-
2 pkts Sweet & Low	4	-	-	-	-	1	-	-	-	-	4.0	-	-	-
2 tbsp Intl creamer	70	-	2.10	-	0	-	.0	12.0	-	.0	10.0	.0	-	.00
1 c fresh pineapple	70	-	2.10	-	0	-	0	17.0	-	2.0	.0	.0	-	.30
2 sl challah	190	-	.12	-	-	90	4.1	40.1	-	-	226.0	82.0	-	1.40
2 vienna finger cookies	130	-	4.50	-	0	-	1.0	22.0	1.0	1.0	105.0	.0	-	.20
1 sl pineapple upside down cake	236	25.0	9.10	-	-	75	2.5	37.4	-	-	179.0	54.0	.41	1.19
2-4 oz 97% FF turkey burgers w/spices	500	-	22.00	H	194	-	72.0	.0	L	-	204.0	-	-	-
1 c grilled vegetables carrots, onions, zucchini, peppers	175	-	.00	-	0	-	7.0	20.0	.0	8.0	60.0	5.0	-	3.00
3 2-inch diameter gingersnap cookies	165	-	10.00	L	10	-	1.0	6.0	L	-	205.0	-	-	-
2 tbsp Cool Whip	25	-	1.50	-	-	-	.0	2.0	1.5	-	.0	-	-	-
8 oz water	-	8.0	-	-	-	-	-	-	-	-	-	-	-	-
DAILY TOTALS	1567	57.0	49.32	0	204	166	87.6	156.5	2.5	11.0	994.0	141.0	.41	6.09

T = trace   H = high   L = low   0 = none   - none   % percent

DAY 80

	Calories 1826 Daily	Fluids	Total Fat 60.90 Daily	Polyunsaturated Fats 20.30 Daily	Cholesterol 300 Daily	Weight Grams	Protein 47.90 Daily	Carbohydrates 264.90 Daily	Saturated Fats 18.27 Daily	Fiber 18.27 Daily	Sodium 1200 Daily	Calcium 1200 Daily	Zinc 13.0 Daily	Iron 10.0 Daily
16 oz water	-	16.0	-	-	-	-	-	-	-	-	-	-	-	-
8 oz decaf coffee	2	8.0	-	-	-	-	-	-	-	-	1.0	-	-	-
2 pkts Sweet & Low	4	-	-	-	-	1	.0	-	-	-	4.0	-	-	-
2 tbsp Intl creamer	70	-	2.1	-	0	-	.0	12.0	-	.00	10.0	.0	-	.00
1 bagel (large)	185	-	4.8	-	-	-	24.0	122.0	-	.24	600.0	8.5	.90	7.20
2 tbsp margarine	150	-	22.0	16.0	0	-	-	-	4.0	-	5.0	-	-	-
1 c Hot Sport energy tea (Ginseng) CF	3	8.0	-	-	-	-	-	2.0	-	-	25.0	-	-	-
1 "Big Mac" hamburger	570	-	35.0	-	83	200	24.6	39.2	-	-	979.0	203.0	-	4.90
17 potato chips	150	-	10.0	-	0	-	2.0	14.0	-	.00	150.0	.0	-	.20
1 c fresh pineapple	70	-	.0	-	-	-	.0	17.0	-	2.00	.0	-	-	.30
3/4 c fresh strawberries	42	132.2	0.5	0.2	0	138	0.8	10.0	.0	2.60	2.0	20.0	.17	.55
8 oz hot water	-	8.0	-	-	-	-	-	-	-	-	-	-	-	-
8 oz cold water	-	8.0	-	-	-	-	-	-	-	-	-	-	-	-
1 slice angel food cake	140	-	.0	-	0	-	3.0	32.0	.0	.00	350.0	.2	-	.20
House visit 2 tbsp onion dip with sour cream	30	-	0.5	-	0	-	1.0	5.0	.0	1.00	610.0	.2	-	.20
17 potato chips	150	-	10.0	-	0	-	2.0	14.0	-	.00	150.0	.0	-	.20
12 oz CF diet Coke	0	12.0	.0	-	-	-	.0	.0	-	-	38.0	-	-	-
1 c Hot Sport energy tea (Ginseng) CF	3	8.0	-	-	-	-	-	2.0	-	-	25.0	-	-	-
2 carrots (raw)	8	-	T	.0	0	-	T	100.0	.0	-	168.0	-	-	-
8 oz water	-	8.0	-	-	-	-	-	-	-	-	-	-	-	-
DAILY TOTALS	1577	208.2	84.9	16.2	83	339	57.4	369.2	4.0	5.84	3117.0	231.9	1.07	13.75

T trace   H high   L low   0 none   - none   % percent

DAY 81

	Calories 1826 Daily	Fluids	Total Fat 60.90 Daily	Polyunsaturated Fats 20.30 Daily	Cholesterol 300 Daily	Weight Grams	Protein 47.90 Daily	Carbohydrates 264.90 Daily	Saturated Fats 18.27 Daily	Fiber 18.27 Daily	Sodium 1200 Daily	Calcium 1200 Daily	Zinc 13.0 Daily	Iron 10.0 Daily
16 oz water	-	16.0	-	-	-	-	-	-	-	-	-	-	-	-
8 oz decaf coffee	2	8.0	T	.0	0	-	T	T	.0	-	1.0	-	-	-
1 bagel (big)	185	-	4.8	-	-	-	24.0	122.0	-	.24	600.0	8.5	.90	7.20
2 pats margarine	150	-	22.0	16.0	.0	-	-	-	4.0	-	5.0	-	-	-
2-1/2 c romaine lettuce	50	-	.1	-	.0	-	2.0	8.0	.0	2.00	.0	.4	-	.40
1/2 c Jello (regular)	80	4.0	.0	-	-	-	2.0	19.0	-	-	80.0	-	-	-
1/2 c sweet red, peppers	12	46.4	.2	.1	.0	50.0	.4	2.7	.0	.60	2.0	3.0	.90	.63
2 tbsp FF low sodium dressing	32	-	.0	-	.0	-	.0	6.0	-	-	280.0	-	-	-
17 potato chips	150	-	10.0	-	.0	-	2.0	14.0	-	.00	150.0	.0	-	.20
2 sl American cheese	420	-	40.0	8.0	90.	100.0	12.30	95.0	10.0	.00	85.0	310.0	1.20	.75
1 sl black forest bread	75	-	1.0	-	.0	-	3.0	15.0	-	1.00	160.0	1.0	-	.50
1 apple (medium)	85	-	T	.5	.1	13.8	.3	21.1	.1	2.80	1.0	10.0	.05	.25
8 oz hot water	-	8.0	-	-	-	-	-	-	-	-	-	-	-	-
1 sl angel food cake	140	-	.0	-	.0	-	3.0	32.0	.0	.00	350.0	.2	-	.20
8 oz water	-	8.0	-	-	-	-	-	-	-	-	-	-	-	-
DAILY TOTALS	1381	90.4	78.1	24.6	90.1	163.8	49.0	334.8	14.1	6.64	1714.0	333.1	3.05	10.13

T = trace   H = high   L = low   0 = none   - none   % percent

DAY 82

	Calories 1826 Daily	Fluids	Total Fat 60.90 Daily	Polyunsaturated Fats 20.30 Daily	Cholesterol 300 Daily	Weight Grams	Protein 47.90 Daily	Carbohydrates 264.90 Daily	Saturated Fats 18.27 Daily	Fiber 18.27 Daily	Sodium 1200 Daily	Calcium 1200 Daily	Zinc 13.0 Daily	Iron 10.0 Daily
16 oz water	-	16.0	-	-	-	-	-	-	-	-	-	-	-	-
8 oz decaf coffee	2	8.0	T	.00	0	-	T	T	.00	-	1.0	-	-	-
2 pkts Sweet & Low	4	-	-	-	-	1	-	-	-	-	4.0	-	-	-
2 tbsp Intl creamer	70	-	2.1	-	0	-	.00	12.0	-	.0	10.0	.0	-	.00
4 oz orange juice	75	4.0	.2	.10	0	128	1.50	12.9	.10	-	1.0	1.4	.60	.25
1 apple cinnamon LF rice cake	50	-	.0	-	-	-	L	10.0	-	-	.0	-	-	-
4 vienna finger cookies	260	-	8.1	-	0	-	2.00	44.0	2.00	2.0	210.0	.0	-	.40
2 sl American cheese	420	-	40.0	8.00	90	100	12.30	95.00	10.00	.0	85.0	310.0	1.20	.75
8 oz hot water	-	8.0	-	-	-	-	-	-	-	-	-	-	-	-
2 raw carrots	8	-	T	.00	0	-	T	50.0	.00	-	84.0	-	-	-
1 big Kosher hot dog	360	-	32.6	.16	70	114	24.18	2.0	24.18	-	1170.0	22.0	2.48	1.40
1 sl black forest bread	75	-	1.0	-	0	-	3.00	15.0	-	1.0	160.0	10.0	.05	.25
2-1/2 c romaine lettuce	50	-	.1	-	0	-	2.00	8.0	.00	2.0	.0	.4	-	.40
8 oz hot sport energy tea (Ginseng) CF	3	8.0	-	-	-	-	-	2.0	-	-	25.0	-	-	-
2 pkts Sweet & Low	4	-	-	-	-	1	-	-	-	-	4.0	-	-	-
4 oz turkey burger	250	-	11.0	H	97	-	34.00	.0	L	-	102.0	-	-	-
1 c grilled vegetables carrots, zucchini, onions, peppers, potatoes	175	-	.0	-	0	-	7.00	20.0	.00	8.0	60.0	5.0	-	3.00
8 oz water	-	8.0	-	-	-	-	-	-	-	-	-	-	-	-
DAILY TOTALS	1806	52.0	95.1	8.26	257	344	85.98	270.9	36.28	13.0	1916.0	348.8	4.33	6.45

T = trace H = high L = low 0 = none - none % percent

	Calories 1826 Daily	Fluids	Total Fat 60.90 Daily	Polyunsaturated Fats 20.30 Daily	Cholesterol 300 Daily	Weight Grams	Protein 47.90 Daily	Carbohydrates 264.90 Daily	Saturated Fats 18.27 Daily	Fiber 18.27 Daily	Sodium 1200 Daily	Calcium 1200 Daily	Zinc 13.0 Daily	Iron 10.0 Daily
16 oz water	-	16.0	-	-	-	-	-	-	-	-	-	-	-	-
8 oz decaf coffee	2	8.0	T	.0	0	-	T	T	.0	-	1.0	-	-	-
2 pkts Sweet & Low	4	-	-	-	-	1.0	-	-	-	-	4.0	-	-	-
2 tbsp Intl creamer	70	-	2.1	-	0	-	.00	12.0	-	.0	10.0	.0	-	.00
1 apple cinnamon LF rice cake	50	-	.0	-	0	-	L	10.0	-	-	.0	-	-	-
1 banana	105	84.7	.6	.1	0	11.4	1.20	26.7	.2	1.6	1.0	7.0	.19	.35
1 "resource" peach yogurt flavored beverage	250	8.0	4.2	-	-	-	8.80	44.4	-	-	65.0	250.0	3.75	4.50
2 tbsp peanut butter	190	.4	16.4	4.1	-	32.0	8.12	4.1	2.8	-	6.0	10.0	.94	.58
9 LF wheat crackers	120	-	-	.0	0	-	.20	21.0	.5	.2	220.0	.2	-	.40
8 oz water	-	8.0	-	-	-	-	-	-	-	-	-	-	-	-
8 oz hot water	-	8.0	-	-	-	-	-	-	-	-	-	-	-	-
1 sl black forest bread	75	-	1.0	-	0	-	3.00	15.0	-	1.0	160.0	10.0	.05	.25
2 tbsp tofu cream cheese	80	-	4.0	6.0	0	-	2.00	2.0	2.0	-	140.0	-	-	-
1/2 c tunafish salad	383	129.5	19.0	8.5	27	205.0	32.90	19.3	3.2	-	824.0	35.0	1.15	2.04
1 c fresh pineapple	70	.0	.0	.0	0	.0	25.00	25.0	.0	3.0	330.0	4.0	-	2.00
8 oz hot sport energy tea (Ginseng) CF	3	8.0	-	-	-	-	-	2.0	-	-	25.0	-	-	-
1 c grilled vegetables sweet peppers, onions zucchini, squash	175	-	.0	-	0	-	7.00	20.0	.0	8.0	60.0	5.0	-	3.00,
8 oz water	-	8.0	-	-	-	-	-	-	-	-	-	-	-	-
DAILY TOTALS	1577	278.6	47.3	18.7	27	249.4	88.22	201.5	8.7	13.8	1846.0	321.2	6.08	13.12

T = trace   H = high   L = low   0 = none   - none   % percent

DAY 84

	Calories 1826 Daily	Fluids	Total Fat 60.90 Daily	Polyunsaturated Fats 20.30 Daily	Cholesterol 300 Daily	Weight Grams	Protein 47.90 Daily	Carbohydrates 264.90 Daily	Saturated Fats 18.27 Daily	Fiber 18.27 Daily	Sodium 1200 Daily	Calcium 1200 Daily	Zinc 13.0 Daily	Iron 10.0 Daily
16 oz water	-	16.0	-	-	-	-	-	-	-	-	-	-	-	-
8 oz decaf coffee	2	8.0	T	.0	0	-	T	T	.0	-	1.0	-	-	-
2 pkts Sweet & Low	4	-	-	-	-	1.0	-	-	-	-	4.0	-	-	-
2 tbsp Intl creamer	70	-	2.1	-	0	-	.0	12.0	-	.00	10.0	.0	-	.00
9 LF wheat crackers	120	-	-	.0	0	-	.2	21.0	2.0	.20	220.0	.2	-	4.00
2 tbsp tofu cream cheese	80	-	4.0	6.0	0	-	2.0	2.0	2.0	-	140.0	-	-	-
1 banana	105	84.7	.6	.1	0	11.4	1.2	26.7	.2	1.60	1.0	7.0	.19	.35
1 bagel (regular)	163	-	2.8	-	-	-	12.0	61.0	10.0	.12	300.0	46.0	.50	3.00
2 sl American cheese	420	-	40.0	8.0	90	100.0	12.30	95.00	10.0	.00	85.0	310.0	1.20	.75
1/2 c tunafish salad w/mayo	400	63.3	14.5	9.3	16	202.0	33.0	19.3	1.0	-	800.0	35.0	1.15	2.04
1/2 c sl Bochusian tomato basil pita bread	100	-	2.0	-	0	-	3.0	18.0	1.0	1.00	200.0	.8	-	.30
8 oz hot sport energy tea (Ginseng) CF	3	8.0	-	-	-	-	-	2.0	-	-	25.0	-	-	-
2 pkts Sweet & Low	4	-	-	-	-	1.0	-	-	-	-	4.0	-	-	-
1c grilled yellow, red sweet peppers	175	-	.0	-	0	-	7.0	20.0	-	8.00	60.0	5.0	-	3.00
8 oz water	-	8.0	-	-	-	-	-	-	-	-	-	-	-	-
DAILY TOTALS	1646	188.0	66.0	23.4	106	315.4	70.7	277.0	19.4	10.92	1850.0	404.0	3.04	13.44

T = trace   H = high   L = low   0 = none   - none   % percent

DAY 85

	Calories 1826 Daily	Fluids	Total Fat 60.90 Daily	Polyunsaturated Fats 20.30 Daily	Cholesterol 300 Daily	Weight Grams	Protein 47.90 Daily	Carbohydrates 264.90 Daily	Saturated Fats 18.27 Daily	Fiber 18.27 Daily	Sodium 1200 Daily	Calcium 1200 Daily	Zinc 13.0 Daily	Iron 10.0 Daily
16 oz water	-	16.0	-	-	-	-	-	-	-	-	-	-	-	-
8 oz decaf coffee	2	8.0	T	.0	0	-	T	T	.0	-	1.0	-	-	-
2 pkts Sweet & Low	4	-	-	-	-	1	-	-	-	-	4.0	-	-	-
2 tbsp Intl creamer	70	-	2.1	-	0	-	.0	12.00	-	.00	10.0	.0	-	.00
2 tbsp tofu cream cheese	80	-	4.0	6.0	0	-	2.0	2.00	2.0	-	140.0	-	-	-
1 bagel (regular)	163	-	2.8	-	-	-	12.0	61.00	-	.12	300.0	46.0	.50	3.00
1 "Big Mac" hamburger	570	-	35.0	-	83	200	24.6	39.20	-	-	979.0	203.0	-	4.90
1 c french fries	300	19.0	18.3	8.8	0	100	4.0	40.00	4.5	.00	216.0	20.0	.38	.76
12 oz CF diet soda	0	12.0	.0	-	-	-	.0	.00	-	-	38.0	-	-	-
1/2 c fruit cocktail	70	4.0	.0	-	0	-	-	17.00	.0	.00	12.0	.0	.00	.00
1 c sweet red peppers	24	92.8	.0	.2	0	100	.8	4.14	.0	.12	4.0	6.0	.158	1.26
5 sl turkey breast	300	68.5	9.6	.2	90	150	58.2	.00	4.0	.00	170.0	30.0	6.10	.09
8 oz water	-	8.0	-	-	-	-	-	-	-	-	-	-	-	-
8 oz hot water	-	8.0	-	-	-	-	-	-	-	-	-	-	-	-
DAILY TOTALS	1583	236.3	72.2	15.2	173	551	101.6	175.34	10.5	.24	1874.0	305.0	7.16	10.01

T = trace   H = high   L = low   0 = none   - none   % percent

DAY 86

	Calories 1826 Daily	Fluids	Total Fat 60.90 Daily	Polyunsaturated Fats 20.30 Daily	Cholesterol 300 Daily	Weight Grams	Protein 47.90 Daily	Carbohydrates 264.90 Daily	Saturated Fats 18.27 Daily	Fiber 18.27 Daily	Sodium 1200 Daily	Calcium 1200 Daily	Zinc 13.0 Daily	Iron 10.0 Daily
16 oz water	-	16.0	-	-	-	-	-	-	-	-	-	-	-	-
8 oz decaf coffee	2	8.0	T	.0	0	-	T	T	.0	-	1.0	-	-	-
2 pkts Sweet & Low	4	-	-	-	-	1	-	-	-	-	4.0	-	-	-
2 tbsp Intl creamer	70	-	2.10	-	0	-	.0	12.0	-	.00	10.0	.0	-	.00
1 bagel (regular)	163	-	2.80	-	-	-	12.0	61.0	-	.12	300.0	46.0	.50	3.00
2 tbsp tofu cream cheese	80	-	4.00	6.0	0	-	2.0	2.0	2.0	-	140.0	-	-	-
2 turkey/hamburg burgers	1172	46.7	39.90	1.0	128	56	40.2	18.8	3.0	3.10	900.0	62.0	-	5.80
2 sl challah	190	-	.12	-	-	90	4.1	40.1	-	-	226.0	82.0	-	1.40
17 potato chips	150	-	10.00	-	0	-	2.0	14.0	-	.00	150.0	.0	-	.20
1 c fresh pineapple	70	-	.00	-	-	-	.0	17.0	-	2.00	.0	-	-	.30
1 c grilled vegetables carrots, squash, onions, zucchini, red, yellow sweet peppers	175	-	.00	-	0	-	7.0	20.0	.0	8.00	60.0	5.0	-	3.00
8 oz water	-	8.0	-	-	-	-	-	-	-	-	-	-	-	-
8 oz hot water	-	8.0	-	-	-	-	-	-	-	-	-	-	-	-
2 vienna fingers	130	-	4.50	-	0	-	1.0	22.0	1.0	1.00	105.0	.0	-	.20
4 oz SF diet Jello	8	4.0	.00	-	0	-	1.0	.0	-	-	50.0	-	-	-
DAILY TOTALS	2214	90.7	63.42	7.0	128	147	69.3	206.9	6.0	14.22	1946.0	195.0	.50	13.90

T = trace   H = high   L = low   0 = none   - none   % percent

	Calories 1826 Daily	Fluids	Total Fat 60.90 Daily	Polyunsaturated Fats 20.30 Daily	Cholesterol 300 Daily	Weight Grams	Protein 47.90 Daily	Carbohydrates 264.90 Daily	Saturated Fats 18.27 Daily	Fiber 18.27 Daily	Sodium 1200 Daily	Calcium 1200 Daily	Zinc 13.0 Daily	Iron 10.0 Daily
16 oz water	-	16.0	-	-	-	-	-	-	-	-	-	-	-	-
8 oz decaf coffee	2	8.0	T	.0	0	-	T	T	.0	-	1.0	-	-	-
2 pkts Sweet & Low	4	-	-	-	-	1	-	-	-	-	4.0	-	-	-
2 tbsp Intl creamer	70	-	2.10	-	0	-	.0	12.00	-	.00	10.0	.0	-	.00
1/2 bagel (regular)	83	-	1.40	-	-	-	6.0	30.90	-	.60	198.0	23.0	.29	1.46
2 tbsp tofu cream cheese	80	-	4.00	6.0	0	-	2.0	2.00	2.0	-	140.0	-	-	-
Wedding Party 3 sl turkey breast	157	66.3	3.20	.9	16	100	29.9	.00	1.0	.00	64.0	19.0	2.04	.02
4 chunks Am cheese	840	-	80.00	169	180	200	24.6	1.90	20.0	.00	170.0	6.2	2.40	1.50
1 c red/yellow sweet peppers	24	92.8	.40	.2	0	100	.8	4.14	.0	.12	4.0	6.0	.18	1.26
9 :F wheat crackers	120	-	-	.0	0	-	.2	21.00	.5	.20	220.0	.2	-	.40
8 oz orange juice	150	8.0	.4	.2	0	256	2.1	24.18	.2	-	2.0	2.8	.12	.50
8 oz water	-	8.0	-	-	-	-	-	-	-	-	-	-	-	
8 oz decaf coffee	2	8.0	T	.0	0	-	T	T	.0	-	1.0	-	-	-
2 tbsp half/half	80	.0	2.14	4.4	12	60	48.2	.12	2.2	.00	12.0	32.0	.16	.02
1 lrg garden salad	150	-	-	-	-	-	-	50.00	-	8.00	3.3	-	-	2.00
1 serving baked fish w/light crumbs	440	-	25.00	.0	0	198	20.0	35.00	.0	.00	640.0	-	-	-
1/2 c string beans	30	-	T	.0	0	-	2.0	6.00	-0	-	6.0	-	-	.10
1 c strawberry ice cream cake w/strawberry syrup	275	-	9.00	.0	0	-	4.0	41.00	.0	-	39.0	176.0	-	.10
3 spinach appetizers	220	-	16.00	-	230	123	12.0	6.00	-	-	365.0	-	-	-
8 oz warm water	-	8.0	-	-	-	-	-	-	-	-	-	-	-	-
DAILY TOTALS	2727	215.1	147.64	27.7	491	1038	151.8	234.24	25.9	8.92	1879.3	265.2	5.19	7.36

T = trace   H = high   L = low   0 = none   - none   % percent

DAY 88

	Calories 1826 Daily	Fluids	Total Fat 60.90 Daily	Polyunsaturated Fats 20.30 Daily	Cholesterol 300 Daily	Weight Grams	Protein 47.90 Daily	Carbohydrates 264.90 Daily	Saturated Fats 18.27 Daily	Fiber 18.27 Daily	Sodium 1200 Daily	Calcium 1200 Daily	Zinc 13.0 Daily	Iron 10.0 Daily
16 oz water	-	16.00	-	-	-	-	-	-	-	-	-	-	-	-
8 oz decaf coffee	2	8.00	T	.0	0	-	T	T	.0	-	1.0	-	-	-
2 pkts Sweet & Low	4	-	-	-	-	1	-	-	-	-	4.0	-	-	-
2 tbsp Intl creamer	70	-	2.10	-	0	-	.0	12.00	-	.00	10.0	.0	-	.00
1 bagel (big)	185	-	4.80	-	-	-	24.0	122.00	-	.24	600.0	8.5	.90	7.20
1 c fresh pineapple	70	-	.00	-	-	-	.0	17.00	-	2.00	.0	-	-	.30
Out for Dinner														
1 lrg garden salad	150	-	-	-	-	-	-	50.00	-	8.00	3.3	-	-	2.0
1 tbsp reg dressing	25	1.10	4.40	2.2	0	7	.0	.20	1.0	-	40.0	.0	.00	.00
16 oz decaf coffee	4	16.00	-	-	-	-	-	-	-	-	2.0	-	-	-
2 pkts Sweet & Low	4	-	-	-	-	1	-	-	-	-	4.0	-	-	-
2 tbsp half/half	80	.00	2.14	4.4	12	60	48.2	.12	2.2	.00	12.0	32.0	.16	.02
1 c grilled vegetables carrots, zucchini, onions	175	-	.00	-	0	-	7.0	20.00	.0	8.0	60.0	5.0	-	3.00
2 sl black forest bread	150	-	2.00	-	0	-	6.0	30.00	-	2.0	320.0	20.0	.10	.50
1/2 c potato salad	210	-	14.00	-	-	113	2.1	18.90	-	-	320.0	21.0	-	1.30
6 oz breaded veal cutlet	230	-	11.00	-	35	142	10.0	20.00	-	-	842.0	66.0	-	1.70
2 pats margarine	150	-	24.00	16.0	0	-	-	-	4.0	-	6.0	-	-	-
8 oz hot water	-	8.00	-	-	-	-	-	-	-	-	-	-	-	-
2 oz jelly beans	208	2.16	.20	-	-	56	.0	32.80	-	-	6.0	6.0	-	.30
8 oz water	-	8.00	-	-	-	-	-	-	-	-	-	-	-	-
DAILY TOTALS	1717	59.26	64.64	22.6	47	380	97.3	323.02	7.2	20.24	2230.3	158.5	1.16	16.32

T = trace   H = high   L = low   0 = none   - none   % percent

DAY 89

	Calories 1826 Daily	Fluids	Total Fat 60.90 Daily	Polyunsaturated Fats 20.30 Daily	Cholesterol 300 Daily	Weight Grams	Protein 47.90 Daily	Carbohydrates 264.90 Daily	Saturated Fats 18.27 Daily	Fiber 18.27 Daily	Sodium 1200 Daily	Calcium 1200 Daily	Zinc 13.0 Daily	Iron 10.0 Daily
16 oz water	-	16.0	-	-	-	-	-	-	-	-	-	-	-	-
8 oz decaf coffee	2	8.0	T	.0	0	-	T	T	.0	-	1.0	-	-	-
2 pkts Sweet & Low	4	-	-	-	-	1.0	-	-	-	-	4.0	-	-	-
2 tbsp Intl creamer	70	-	2.1	-	0	-	.0	12.00	-	.00	10.0	.0	-	.00
1/2 bagel (regular)	83	-	1.4	-	-	-	6.0	30.90	-	.60	198.0	23.0	.29	1.46
2 tbsp tofu cream cheese	80	-	4.0	6.0	0	-	2.0	2.00	2.0	-	140.0	-	-	-
1 banana	105	84.7	.6	.1	0	11.4	1.2	26.70	.2	1.60	1.0	7.0	.19	.35
1/2 c green grapes	58	14.8	.3	.1	0	92.0	.6	15.80	.1	.00	2.0	13.0	.04	.27
3 oz roast chicken	142	-	6.0	H	80	-	35.0	.00	L	.00	87.0	12.0	.00	1.70
1 c yellow sweet peppers	24	92.8	.4	.2	0	100.0	.8	4.14	.0	.12	4.0	6.0	.18	1.26
8 oz Crystal Light	6	8.0	.0	.0	0	-	.0	.10	-	.00	.0	.0	.00	.00
1 sl black forest bread	75	-	1.0	-	0	-	3.0	15.00	-	1.00	160.0	10.0	.05	.25
8 oz hot water	-	8.0	-	-	-	-	-	-	-	-	-	-	-	-
8 oz water	-	8.0	-	-	-	-	-	-	-	-	-	-	-	-
DAILY TOTALS	649	240.3	15.8	6.4	80	204.4	48.6	106.64	2.3	3.32	607.0	71.0	.75	5.29

T = trace   H = high   L = low   0 = none   - none   % percent

DAY 90

	Calories 1826 Daily	Fluids	Total Fat 60.90 Daily	Polyunsaturated Fats 20.30 Daily	Cholesterol 300 Daily	Weight Grams	Protein 47.90 Daily	Carbohydrates 264.90 Daily	Saturated Fats 18.27 Daily	Fiber 18.27 Daily	Sodium 1200 Daily	Calcium 1200 Daily	Zinc 13.0 Daily	Iron 10.0 Daily
16 oz water	-	16.0	-	-	-	-	-	-	-	-	-	-	-	-
8 oz decaf coffee	2	8.0	T	.0	0	-	T	T	.0	-	1.0	-	-	-
2 pkts Sweet & Low	4	-	-	-	-	1	-	-	-	-	4.0	-	-	-
2 tbsp Intl creamer	70	-	2.1	-	0	-	.0	12.0	-	.0	10.0	.0	-	.00
1/2 c fruit cocktail	70	4.0	.0	-	0	-	-	17.0	.0	.0	12.0	.0	.00	.00
1 Dunkin Donut (honey dip, same as jelly)	245	-	10.0	T	30	-	3.0	37.0	6.8	-	143.0	-	-	-
8 oz decaf coffee	2	8.0	T	.0	0	-	T	T	.0	-	1.0	-	-	-
2 tbsp milk (regular)	50	2.0	6.0	.0	16	-	4.0	8.0	.8	.2	80.0	2.1	-	.20
2 pkts Sweet & Low	4	-	-	-	-	1	-	-	-	-	4.0	-	-	-
3 oz roast chicken	142	-	6.0	H	80	-	35.0	.0	L	.0	87.0	12.0	.00	1.70
1/2 c diet Jello	8	4.0	.0	-	0	-	1.0	.0	-	-	50.0	-	-	-
1 c mashed potatoes w/crumbs	111	80.1	4.4	1.3	2	105	2.0	17.5	1.1	.0	309.0	27.0	.29	.28
2 pats margarine	150	-	22.0	16.0	0	-	-	-	4.0	-	5.0	-	-	-
8 oz Crystal Light	6	8.0	.0	.0	0	-	.0	.1	-	.0	.0	.0	.00	.00
8 oz hot water	-	8.0	-	-	-	-	-	-	-	-	-	-	-	-
8 oz water	-	8.0	-	-	-	-	-	-	-	-	-	-	-	-
DAILY TOTALS	864	146.1	50.5	17.3	128	107	45.0	91.6	12.7	.2	706.0	41.1	.29	2.18

T = trace   H = high   L = low   0 = none   - none   % percent

DAY 91

	Calories 1826 Daily	Fluids	Total Fat 60.90 Daily	Polyunsaturated Fats 20.30 Daily	Cholesterol 300 Daily	Weight Grams	Protein 47.90 Daily	Carbohydrates 264.90 Daily	Saturated Fats 18.27 Daily	Fiber 18.27 Daily	Sodium 1200 Daily	Calcium 1200 Daily	Zinc 13.0 Daily	Iron 10.0 Daily
16 oz water	-	16.0	-	-	-	-	-	-	-	-	-	-	-	-
8 oz decaf coffee	2	8.0	T	.0	0	-	T	T	.0	-	1.0	-	-	-
2 pkts Sweet & Low	4	-	-	-	-	1	-	-	-	-	4.0	-	-	-
2 tbsp Intl creamer	70	-	2.1	-	0	-	.0	12.0	-	.0	10.0	.0	-	.00
1 "Big Mac" hamburger	570	-	35.0	-	83	200	24.6	39.2	-	-	979.0	203.0	-	4.90
1 c french fries	300	19.0	18.3	8.8	0	100	4.0	40.0	4.5	.0	216.0	20.0	.38	.76
1/2 c cauliflower	12	46.1	.1	.0	0	50	1.0	2.5	.0	-	7.0	14.0	.09	.29
1 tbsp reg dressing	25	1.1	4.4	2.2	0	7	.0	.2	1.0	-	40.0	.0	.00	.00
1 c tunafish salad w/light mayo	800	129.5	29.0	18.5	37	405	65.0	38.6	6.4	-	1600.0	70.0	2.30	4.08
8 oz water	-	8.0	-	-	-	-	-	-	-	-	-	-	-	-
12 oz CF diet Coke	0	12.0	.0	-	-	-	.0	.0	-	-	38.0	-	-	-
8 oz hot water	-	8.0	-	-	-	-	-	-	-	-	-	-	-	-
2 pkts Sweet & Low	4	-	-	-	-	1	-	-	-	-	4.0	-	-	-
8 oz water	-	8.0	-	-	-	-	-	-	-	-	-	-	-	-
DAILY TOTALS	1787	255.7	88.9	29.5	120	764	94.6	132.5	11.9	.0	2899.0	307.0	2.77	10.03

T = trace   H = high   L = low   0 = none   - none   % percent

DAY 92

	Calories 1826 Daily	Fluids	Total Fat 60.90 Daily	Polyunsaturated Fats 20.30 Daily	Cholesterol 300 Daily	Weight Grams	Protein 47.90 Daily	Carbohydrates 264.90 Daily	Saturated Fats 18.27 Daily	Fiber 18.27 Daily	Sodium 1200 Daily	Calcium 1200 Daily	Zinc 13.0 Daily	Iron 10.0 Daily
16 oz water	-	16.0	-	-	-	-	-	-	-	-	-	-	-	-
8 oz decaf coffee	2	8.0	T	.0	0	-	T	T	.0	-	1.0	-	-	-
2 tbsp milk	50	2.0	6.00	.0	16	-	4.0	8.00	.8	.2	80.0	2.1	-	.20
2 pkts Sweet & Low	4	-	-	-	-	1	-	-	-	-	4.0	-	-	-
1/2 bagel	83	-	1.40	-	-	-	6.0	30.90	-	.6	198.0	23.0	.29	1.46
2 tbsp FF cream cheese	30	-	.00	-	1	-	4.0	3.00	.0	.0	150.0	6.0	-	.00
2-1/2 c romaine lettuce	50	-	.10	-	0	-	2.0	8.00	.0	2.0	.0	.4	-	.40
1 tbsp reg dressing	25	1.1	4.40	2.2	0	7	.0	.20	1.0	-	40.0	.0	.00	.00
1/2 c cauliflower	12	46.1	.10	.0	0	50	1.0	2.50	.0	-	7.0	14.0	.09	.29
8 oz water	-	8.0	-	-	-	-	-	-	-	-	-	-	-	-
Out for Dinner														
1 garden salad	150	-	-	-	-	-	-	50.00	-	8.0	3.3	-	-	2.00
1 tbsp reg dressing	25	1.1	4.40	2.2	0	7	.0	.20	1.0	-	40.0	.0	.00	.00
24 oz decaf coffee	12	24.0	-	-	-	-	-	-	-	6.0	-	-	-	-
4 pkts Sweet & Low	8	-	-	-	-	3	-	-	-	-	8.0	-	-	-
5 tbsp half/half	160	.0	4.28	8.8	24	120	96.4	.24	4.4	.0	24.0	64.0	.32	.04
1/2 c potato salad	210	-	14.00	-	-	113	2.1	18.90	-	-	320.0	21.0	-	1.30
1 sl black forest bread	75	-	1.00	-	0	-	3.0	15.00	-	1.0	160.0	10.0	.05	.25
2 pats margarine	150	-	24.00	16.0	0	-	-	-	4.0	-	6.0	-	-	-
1 c french fries	300	19.0	18.30	8.8	0	100	4.0	40.00	4.5	.0	216.0	20.0	.38	.76
1 "Ruben on Rye" (lean) sandwich	512	-	31.40	-	105	194	30.1	39.40	-	-	1224.0	237.0	5.23	.43
8 oz water	-	8.0	-	-	-	-	-	-	-	-	-	-	-	-
DAILY TOTALS	1858	141.3	113.38	38.0	146	595	152.6	216.34	15.7	17.8	2481.3	397.5	6.36	7.13

T = trace   H = high   L = low   0 = none   - none   % percent

DAY 93

	Calories 1,826 Daily	Fluids	Total Fat 60.90 Daily	Polyunsaturated Fats 20.30 Daily	Cholesterol 300 Daily	Weight Grams	Protein 47.90 Daily	Carbohydrates 264.90 Daily	Saturated Fats 18.27 Daily	Fiber 18.27 Daily	Sodium 1200 Daily	Calcium 1200 Daily	Zinc 13.0 Daily	Iron 10.0 Daily
16 oz water	-	16.0	-	-	-	-	-	-	-	-	-	-	-	-
8 oz decaf coffee	2	8.0	T	.0	0	-	T	T	.0	-	1.0	-	-	-
2 pkts Sweet & Low	4	-	-	-	-	1	-	-	-	-	4.0	-	-	-
2 tbsp Intl creamer	70	-	2.1	-	0	-	.0	12.00	-	.0	10.0	.0	-	.00
1/2 c chicken salad	90	-	4.6	-	16	56	8.4	2.16	-	-	156.0	10.0	-	6.80
2 raw carrots	8	-	T	.0	0	-	T	50.00	.0	-	84.0	-	-	-
12 oz CF diet Coke	0	12.0	.0	-	-	-	.0	.00	-	-	38.0	-	-	-
1 Dunkin Donut honey dipped (same as jelly)	245	-	10.0	T	30	-	3.0	37.00	6.8	-	143.0	-	-	-
Out for Dinner 6 oz breaded veal cutlet	230	-	11.0	-	35	142	10.0	20.00	-	-	842.0	66.0	-	1.70
16 oz water	-	16.0	-	-	-	-	-	-	-	-	-	-	-	-
2 sl black forest bread	150	-	2.0	-	0	-	6.0	30.00	-	2.0	320.0	20.0	.10	.50
2 pats margarine	150	-	24.0	16.0	0	-	-	-	4.0	-	6.0	-	-	-
1 lrg garden salad	150	-	-	-	-	-	-	50.00	-	8.0	3.3	-	-	2.0
8 oz hot water	-	8.0	-	-	-	-	-	-	-	-	-	-	-	-
8 oz water	-	8.0	-	-	-	-	-	-	-	-	-	-	-	-
DAILY TOTALS	1099	68.0	53.7	16.0	81	199	27.4	201.16	10.8	10.0	1607.3	96.0	.10	11.00

T = trace   H = high   L = low   0 = none   - none   % percent

	Calories 1826 Daily	Fluids	Total Fat 60.90 Daily	Polyunsaturated Fats 20.30 Daily	Cholesterol 300 Daily	Weight Grams	Protein 47.90 Daily	Carbohydrates 264.90 Daily	Saturated Fats 18.27 Daily	Fiber 18.27 Daily	Sodium 1200 Daily	Calcium 1200 Daily	Zinc 13.0 Daily	Iron 10.0 Daily
16 oz water	-	16.0	-	-	-	-	-	-	-	-	-	-	-	-
8 oz decaf coffee	2	8.0	T	.0	0	-	T	T	.0	-	1.00	-	-	-
2 pkts Sweet & Low	4	-	-	-	-	1	-	-	-	-	4.00	-	-	-
2 tbsp Intl creamer	70	-	2.1	-	0	-	.0	12.00	-	.00	10.00	.0	-	.00
1 large bagel	185	-	4.8	-	-	-	24.0	122.00	-	.24	600.00	8.5	.90	7.20
2 tbsp FF cream cheese	30	-	.0	-	1	-	4.0	3.00	.0	.00	150.00	6.0	-	.00
5 sl turkey breast	300	68.5	9.6	.2	90	150	58.2	.00	4.0	.00	170.00	30.0	6.10	.09
1 c sweet red and yellow peppers	24	92.8	.4	.2	0	100	.8	4.14	.0	.12	4.00	6.0	.18	1.26
4 oz water	-	4.0	-	-	-	-	-	-	-	-	-	-	-	-
$1/2$ of a cucumber	7	-	.1	.0	0	52	.3	1.50	.0	.30	1.00	7.0	.12	.21
12 oz CF diet Coke	0	12.0	.0	-	-	-	.0	.00	-	-	38.00	-	-	-
Out for Supper														
12 oz CF diet Coke	0	12.0	.0	-	-	-	.0	.00	-	-	38.00	-	-	-
4 sl cheese pizza	960	-	36.0	T	120	-	56.0	100.00	T	2114.00	4.16	-	-	
8 oz hot water	-	8.0	-	-	-	-	-	-	-	-	-	-	-	-
8 oz water	-	8.0	-	-	-	-	-	-	-	-	-	-	-	-
DAILY TOTALS	1582	229.3	53.0	.4	211	303	143.3	242.64	4.0	2114.66	1020.16	57.5	7.30	8.76

T = trace   H = high   L = low   0 = none   - none   % percent

DAY 95

	Calories 1826 Daily	Fluids	Total Fat 60.90 Daily	Polyunsaturated Fats 20.30 Daily	Cholesterol 300 Daily	Weight Grams	Protein 47.90 Daily	Carbohydrates 264.90 Daily	Saturated Fats 18.27 Daily	Fiber 18.27 Daily	Sodium 1200 Daily	Calcium 1200 Daily	Zinc 13.0 Daily	Iron 10.0 Daily
16 oz water	-	16.0	-	-	-	-	-	-	-	-	-	-	-	-
8 oz decaf coffee	2	8.0	T	.0	0	-	T	T	.0	-	1.0	-	-	-
2 pkts Sweet & Low	4	-	-	-	-	1	-	-	-	-	4.0	-	-	-
2 tbsp Intl creamer	70	-	2.1	-	0	-	.0	12.00	-	.00	10.0	.0	-	.00
1 c cantaloupe	57	143.6	.4	-	-	160	1.4	13.40	-	.50	14.0	17.0	.25	.34
1 cinnamon apple LF rice cake	50	-	.0	-	0	-	1.0	11.00	-	-	.0	-	-	-
5 sl turkey breast	300	68.5	9.6	.2	90	150	58.2	.00	4.0	.00	170.0	30.0	6.10	.09
1 c red and yellow sweet peppers	24	92.8	.4	.2	0	100	.8	4.14	.0	.12	4.0	6.0	.18	1.26
1 c pineapple	70	-	.0	-	-	-	.0	17.00	-	2.00	.0	-	-	.30
8 oz water	-	8.0	-	-	-	-	-	-	-	-	-	-	-	-
2-servings (2x2) noodle pudding	390	-	26.0	T	60	-	18.0	20.00	H	-	400.0	40.0	-	.20
1 c canned vegetable soup	70	-	1.5	-	-	2.1	2.8	12.10	-	-	730.0	21.0	-	1.50
8 oz hot water	-	8.0	-	-	-	-	-	-	-	-	-	-	-	-
1/2 bagel	83	-	1.4	-	-	-	6.0	30.90	-	.60	198.0	23.0	.29	1.46
2 pages margarine	150	-	24.0	16.0	0	-	-	-	4.0	-	6.0	-	-	-
8 oz water	-	8.0	-	-	-	-	-	-	-	-	-	-	-	-
DAILY TOTALS	1270	352.9	65.4	16.4	150	412.1	88.2	120.54	8.0	3.22	1537.0	137.0	6.82	5.15

T = trace   H = high   L = low   0 = none   - none   % percent

DAY 96

	Calories 1826 Daily	Fluids	Total Fat 60.90 Daily	Polyunsaturated Fats 20.30 Daily	Cholesterol 300 Daily	Weight Grams	Protein 47.90 Daily	Carbohydrates 264.90 Daily	Saturated Fats 18.27 Daily	Fiber 18.27 Daily	Sodium 1200 Daily	Calcium 1200 Daily	Zinc 13.0 Daily	Iron 10.0 Daily
16 oz water	-	16.0	-	-	-	-	-	-	-	-	-	-	-	-
8 oz decaf coffee	2	8.0	T	.0	0	-	T	T	.0	-	1.0	-	-	-
2 pkts Sweet & Low	4	-	-	-	-	1	-	-	-	-	4.0	-	-	-
2 tbsp Intl creamer	70	-	2.10	-	0	-	.0	12.0	-	.0	10.0	.0	-	.000
4 oz 1% milk	55	4.0	1.40	-	12	-	4.0	9.0	1.0	.0	-	25.0	-	.000
2 sm boxes Grainfield raisin bran cereal	2200	-	1.05	-	0	0	.0	43.0	.0	6.0	20.0	.1	-	.800
8 graham crackers	480	.3	8.90	-	-	94	8.0	80.9	-	-	550.0	30.0	.88	.136
4 oz orange juice	75	4.0	.20	.1	0	128	1.5	12.9	.1	-	1.0	1.4	.60	.250
8 oz water	-	8.0	-	-	-	-	-	-	-	-	-	-	-	-
1/2 c pc Bochusian tomato basil pita bread	100	-	2.00	-	0	-	3.00	18.0	1.0	1.0	200.0	.8	-	.300
2 c orange sweet peppers	316	-	.00	-	0	-	12.0	20.0	.0	12.0	118.0	12.0	-	4.100
1 c roasted potatoes	157	154.4	2.50	.1	7	194	4.6	30.0	1.5	-	421.0	70.0	.59	.910
8 oz hot water	-	8.0	-	-	-	-	-	-	-	-	-	-	-	-
8 oz water	-	8.0	-	-	-	-	-	-	-	-	-	-	-	-
DAILY TOTALS	1479	210.7	18.15	.2	19	417	33.1	225.8	3.6	19.0	1325.0	139.3	2.07	6.496

T = trace   H = high   L = low   0 = none   - none   % percent

DAY 97

	Calories 1826 Daily	Fluids	Total Fat 60.90 Daily	Polyunsaturated Fats 20.30 Daily	Cholesterol 300 Daily	Weight Grams	Protein 47.90 Daily	Carbohydrates 264.90 Daily	Saturated Fats 18.27 Daily	Fiber 18.27 Daily	Sodium 1200 Daily	Calcium 1200 Daily	Zinc 13.0 Daily	Iron 10.0 Daily
16 oz water	-	16.00	-	-	-	-	-	-	-	-	-	-	-	-
8 oz decaf coffee	2	8.00	T	.0	0	-	T	T	.0	-	1.0	-	-	-
2 pkts Sweet & Low	4	-	-	-	-	1	-	-	-	-	4.0	-	-	-
2 tbsp Intl creamer	70	-	2.1	-	0	-	.00	12.00	-	.0	10.0	.0	-	.00
2 c orange sweet peppers	316	-	.0	-	0	-	12.00	20.00	.0	12.0	118.0	12.0	-	4.10
1 c seedless green grapes	116	28.16	.6	.2	0	184	.120	30.16	.2	.0	4.0	26.0	.08	.54
12 oz CF diet coke	0	12.00	.0	-	-	-	.00	.00	-	-	38.0	-	-	-
3 vanilla wafers	110	.50	1.1	-	-	28	1.50	25.00	-	1.0	203.0	8.0	2.25	4.50
3 graham crackers	260	.10	3.3	-	-	45	4.00	40.20	-	-	325.0	2.0	.42	.75
2 fried egg whites	20	.00	1.0	.0	0	0	6.00	.00	.0	-	45.0	.0	.00	.00
2 c yellow sweet peppers	316	-	.0	-	0	-	12.00	20.00	.0	12.0	118.0	12.0	-	4.10
1 c grilled vegetables onions, tomatoes, zucchini, squash	150	-	.0	-	0	-	4.00	9.00	.0	4.0	50.0	4.0	-	2.00
8 oz hot water	-	8.00	-	-	-	-	-	-	-	-	-	-	-	-
8 oz hot water	-	8.00	-	-	-	-	-	-	-	-	-	-	-	-
DAILY TOTALS	1364	80.76	8.1	.2	0	258	39.62	156.36	.2	29.0	916.0	64.0	2.75	15.99

T = trace   H = high   L = low   0 = none   - none   % percent

	Calories 1826 Daily	Fluids	Total Fat 60.90 Daily	Polyunsaturated Fats 20.30 Daily	Cholesterol 300 Daily	Weight Grams	Protein 47.90 Daily	Carbohydrates 264.90 Daily	Saturated Fats 18.27 Daily	Fiber 18.27 Daily	Sodium 1200 Daily	Calcium 1200 Daily	Zinc 13.0 Daily	Iron 10.0 Daily
16 oz water	-	16.0	-	-	-	-	-	-	-	-	-	-	-	-
8 oz decaf coffee	2	8.0	T	.0	0	-	T	T	.0	-	1.0	-	-	-
2 pkts Sweet & Low	4	-	-	-	-	1	-	-	-	-	4.0	-	-	-
2 tbsp Intl creamer	70	-	2.1	-	0	-	.0	12.0	-	.0	10.0	.0	-	.00
4 oz orange juice	75	4.0	.2	.1	0	128	1.5	12.9	.1	-	1.0	1.4	.60	.25
1 yogurt flavored nutrition drink	250	8.0	4.2	-	-	-	8.8	44.4	-	-	65.0	250.0	3.75	4.50
4 raw carrots	16	-	T	.0	0	-	T	100.00	.0	-	168.0	-	-	-
4 oatmeal/raisin cookies	235	1.5	8.0	-	-	52	3.2	38.2	2.1	-	84	11.0	-	1.50
2 sl French pametta bread	120		.0	-	0	-	4.0	24.0	.0	1.0	310.0	.0	-	.60
2 pats margarine	150	-	22.0	16.0	0	-	-	-	4.0	-	5.0	-	-	-
1 serving beef stir fry meatballs, red peppers, green beans carrots, noodles	260	-	6.0	-	65	255	24.0	27.0	-	-	790.0	45.0	-	3.00
8 oz water	-	8.0	-	-	-	-	-	-	-	-	-	-	-	-
8 oz Crystal Light	6	8.0	.0	.0	0	-	.0	.1	-	.0	.0	.0	.00	.00
¼ c cantaloupe	52	160.2	.4	-	0	160	2.0	12.6	-	.2	14.0	18.0	.26	.30
8 oz hot water	-	8.0	-	-	-	-	-	-	-	-	-	-	-	-
DAILY TOTALS	1240	221.7	42.9	16.1	65	596	43.5	271.2	6.2	1.2	1452.0	325.4	4.61	10.15

T = trace   H = high   L = low   0 = none   - none   % percent

DAY 99

	Calories 1826 Daily	Fluids	Total Fat 60.90 Daily	Polyunsaturated Fats 20.30 Daily	Cholesterol 300 Daily	Weight Grams	Protein 47.90 Daily	Carbohydrates 264.90 Daily	Saturated Fats 18.27 Daily	Fiber 18.27 Daily	Sodium 1200 Daily	Calcium 1200 Daily	Zinc 13.0 Daily	Iron 10.0 Daily
16 oz water	-	16.0	-	-	-	-	-	-	-	-	-	-	-	-
8 oz decaf coffee	2	8.0	T	.0	0	-	T	T	.0	-	1.0	-	-	-
2 pkts Sweet & Low	4	-	-	-	-	1	-	-	-	-	4.0	-	-	-
2 tbsp Intl creamer	70	-	2.1	-	0	-	.0	12.00	-	.0	10.0	.00	-	.00
4 oz orange/tangerine juice	60	4.0	.0	-	0	-	.0	27.00	-	-	14.0	.35	-	-
3 fig squares	225	-	4.0		0	-	2.0	39.00	2.0	.0	270.0	.00	.00	.20
1 sl American cheese	210	-	20.0	4.0	45	50	6.1	45.00	5.0	.0	42.0	1.15	1.00	.35
1 c yellow sweet peppers	24	92.8	.4	.2	0	100	.8	4.14	.0	.12	4.0	6.00	.18	1.26
1 scone (plain)	270	-	9.0	-	10	-	-	41.00	-	2.0	610.0	4.00	-	.10
1/2 c tunafish salad	383	129.5	19.0	8.5	27	205	32.9	19.30	3.2	-	824.0	35.00	1.15	2.04
8 oz hot sport energy tea (Ginseng) CF	3	8.0	-	-	-	-	-	2.00	-	-	25.0	-	-	-
12 oz CF diet coke	0	12.0	.0	-	-	-	.0	.00	-	-	38.0	-	-	-
8 oz water	-	8.0	-	-	-	-	-	-	-	-	-	-	-	-
DAILY TOTALS	1251	278.3	54.5	12.7	82	356	41.8	189.44	10.2	2.12	1842.0	46.50	2.33	3.95

T = trace   H = high   L = low   0 = none   - none   % percent

DAY 100

	Calories 1826 Daily	Fluids	Total Fat 60.90 Daily	Polyunsaturated Fats 20.30 Daily	Cholesterol 300 Daily	Weight Grams	Protein 47.90 Daily	Carbohydrates 264.90 Daily	Saturated Fats 18.27 Daily	Fiber 18.27 Daily	Sodium 1200 Daily	Calcium 1200 Daily	Zinc 13.0 Daily	Iron 10.0 Daily
16 oz water	-	16.0	-	-	-	-	-	-	-	-	-	-	-	-
8 oz decaf coffee	2	8.0	T	.00	0	-	T	T	.0	-	1.0	-	-	-
2 pkts Sweet & Low	4	-	-	-	-	1	-	-	-	-	4.0	-	-	-
2 tbsp Intl creamer	70	-	2.1	-	0	-	.0	12.00	-	.00	10.0	.0	-	.00
3 fig squares	225	-	4.0	-	0	-	2.0	39.00	2.0	.00	270.0	.0	.00	.20
Out for Lunch 1 English muffin w/butter	186	-	5.3	-	15	63.0.0	5.0	29.50	-	-	310.0	117.0	-	1.51
2 fried egg whites	20	.0	1.0	.00	0	.0	6.0	.00	.0	-	45.0	.0	.00	.00
1 sl crisp bacon	43	14.3	2.2	.20	16	2.4	6.1	.30	1.0	.00	300.0	3.0	.41	.24
1 c home fries	316	38.0	16.6	6.16	0	100.0	4.0	40.00	4.1	-	216.0	20.0	.38	.76
4 oz corn beef hash	145	-	7.0	L	60	-	16.0	8.00	H	-	612.0	-	-	-
16 oz decaf coffee	4	16.0	T	.00	0	-	T	T	.0	-	2.0	-	-	-
2 pkts Sweet & Low	4	-	-	-	-	1.0	-	-	-	-	4.0	-	-	-
3 cntnrs half/half	120	.0	2.1	6.80	18	90.0	88.3	.18	2.2	.00	18.0	36.0	.24	.03
2 tbsp FF dressing	45	-	.0	.00	0	.0	.0	11.00	.0	1.00	330.0	.0	.00	.00
1 lrg garden salad	150	-	-	-	-	-	-	50.00	-	8.00	3.3	-	-	2.00
1 c yellow sweet pepper	24	92.8	.4	.20	0	100.0	.8	4.14	.0	.12	4.0	6.0	.18	1.26
1 c fresh pineapple	70	-	.0	-	-	-	.0	17.00	-	2.00	.0	-	-	3.00
16 oz water	-	16.0	-	-	-	-	-	-	-	-	-	-	-	-
8 oz hot water	-	8.0	-	-	-	-	-	-	-	-	-	-	-	-
DAILY TOTALS	1428	209.1	40.7	13.36	109	357.4	128.2	211.12	9.3	11.12	2129.3	182.0	1.21	9.29

T = trace   H = high   L = low   0 = none   - none   % percent

	Calories 1826 Daily	Fluids	Total Fat 60.90 Daily	Polyunsaturated Fats 20.30 Daily	Cholesterol 300 Daily	Weight Grams	Protein 47.90 Daily	Carbohydrates 264.90 Daily	Saturated Fats 18.27 Daily	Fiber 18.27 Daily	Sodium 1200 Daily	Calcium 1200 Daily	Zinc 13.0 Daily	Iron 10.0 Daily
DAILY TOTALS														

T = trace   H = high   L = low   0 = none   - none   % percent

* amount exaggerated